I0100857

Llama Locomotion

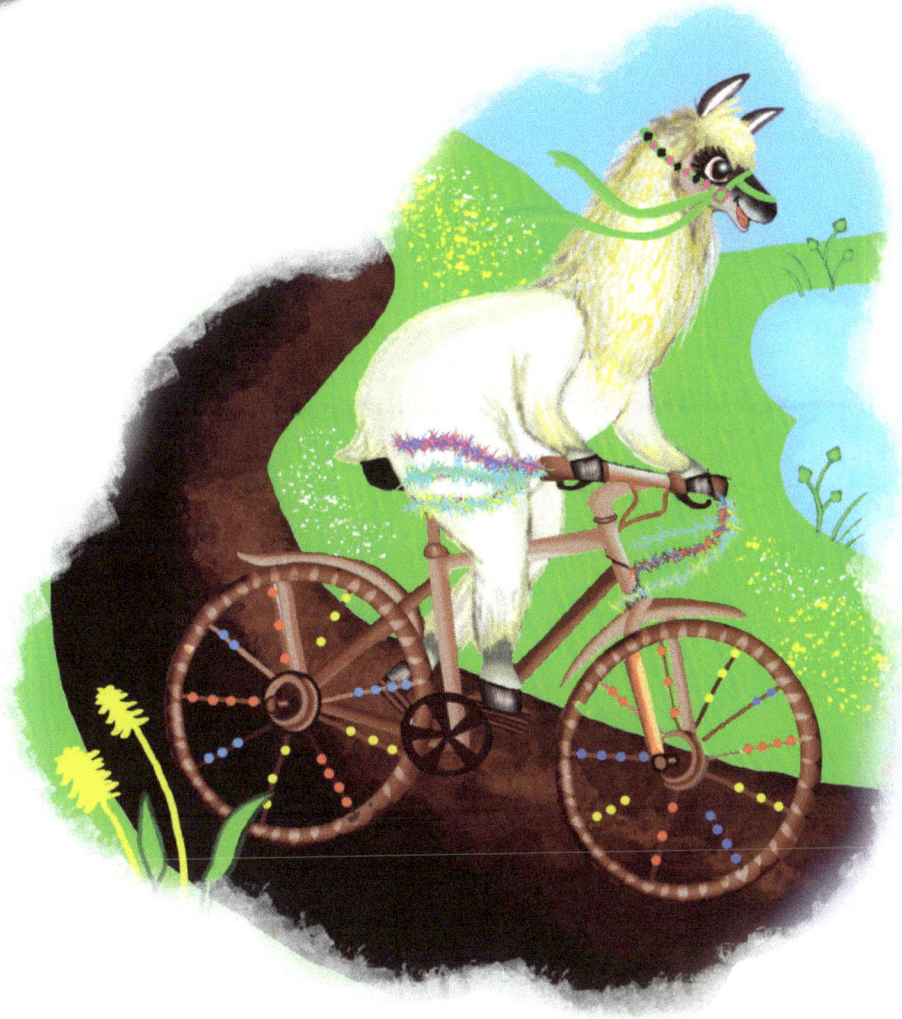

Written by Dr. Deborah Sharp Molchan

Illustrated by Emily Hercock

Copyright 2022 by Oprelle Publications

Paperback ISBN: 979-8-9857483-0-7
First printing edition 2022

Written by Deborah Sharp Molchan
Illustrated by Emily Hercock

All rights reserved. No part of this publication may be reproduced, distributed or transmitted in any form or by any means, including photocopying, recording, or other electronic or mechanical methods, without the prior written permission of the publisher, except in the case of brief quotations embodied in critical reviews and certain other noncommercial uses permitted by copyright law.

To my husband, David, and my daughters, Kate and Lauren:

You are forever my favorite Llama Locomotion playmates.

Love you forever.

- D.S.M.

"Mama Llama, my thoughts rush like a speeding train.
My racing thoughts ache my brain.

My llama legs wiggle and want to play.
Llamas don't sit still all day."

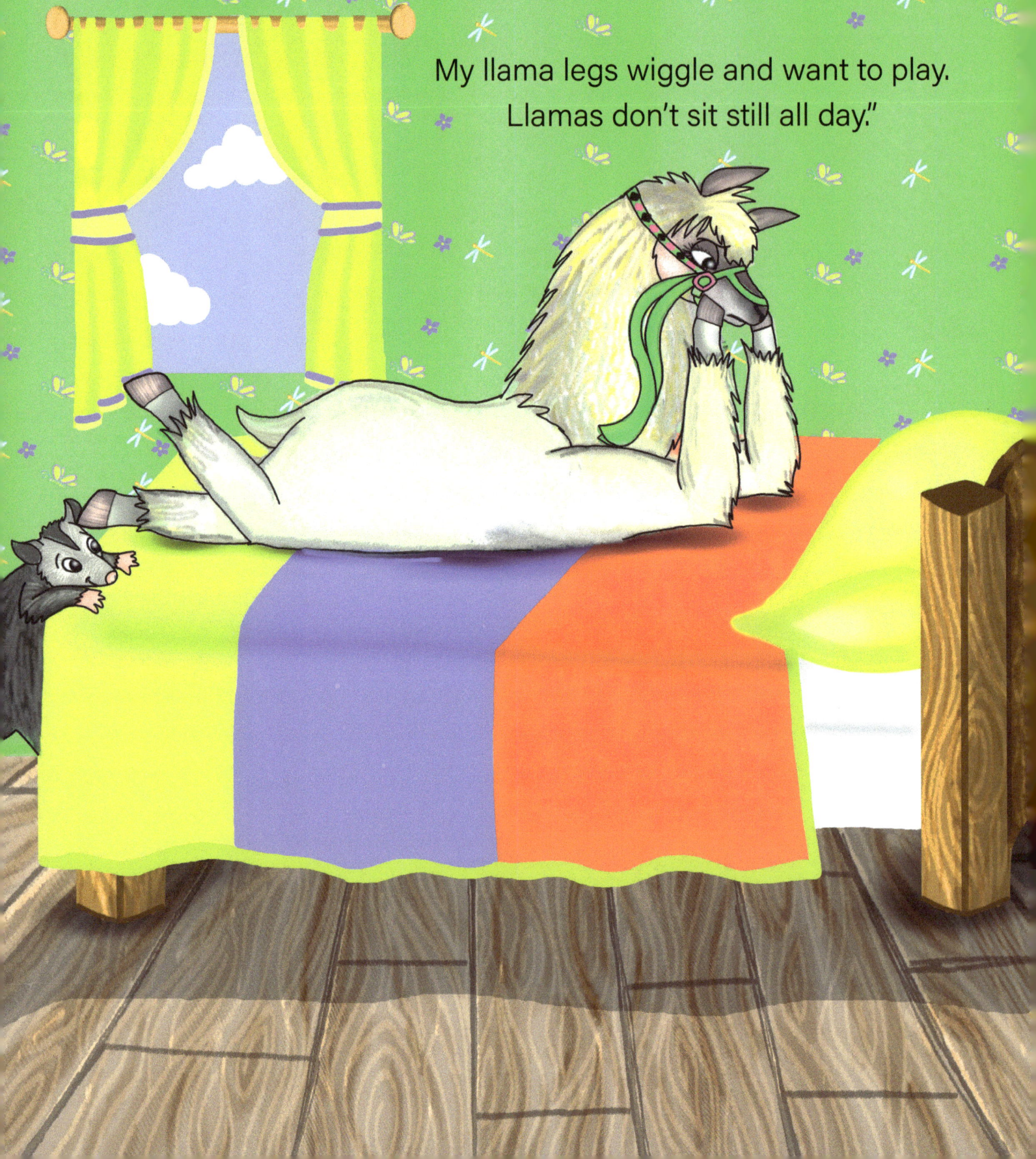

"Sammy," Mama Llama said, "Get up and bike, move your mood.

Bike with Stan; it's great brain food."

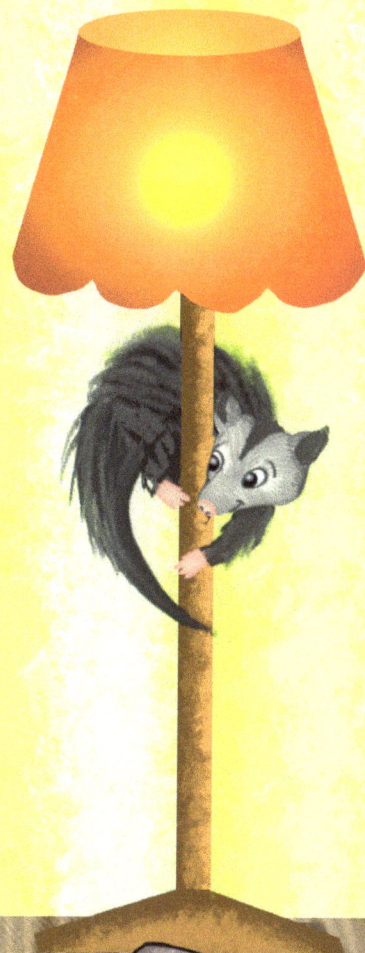

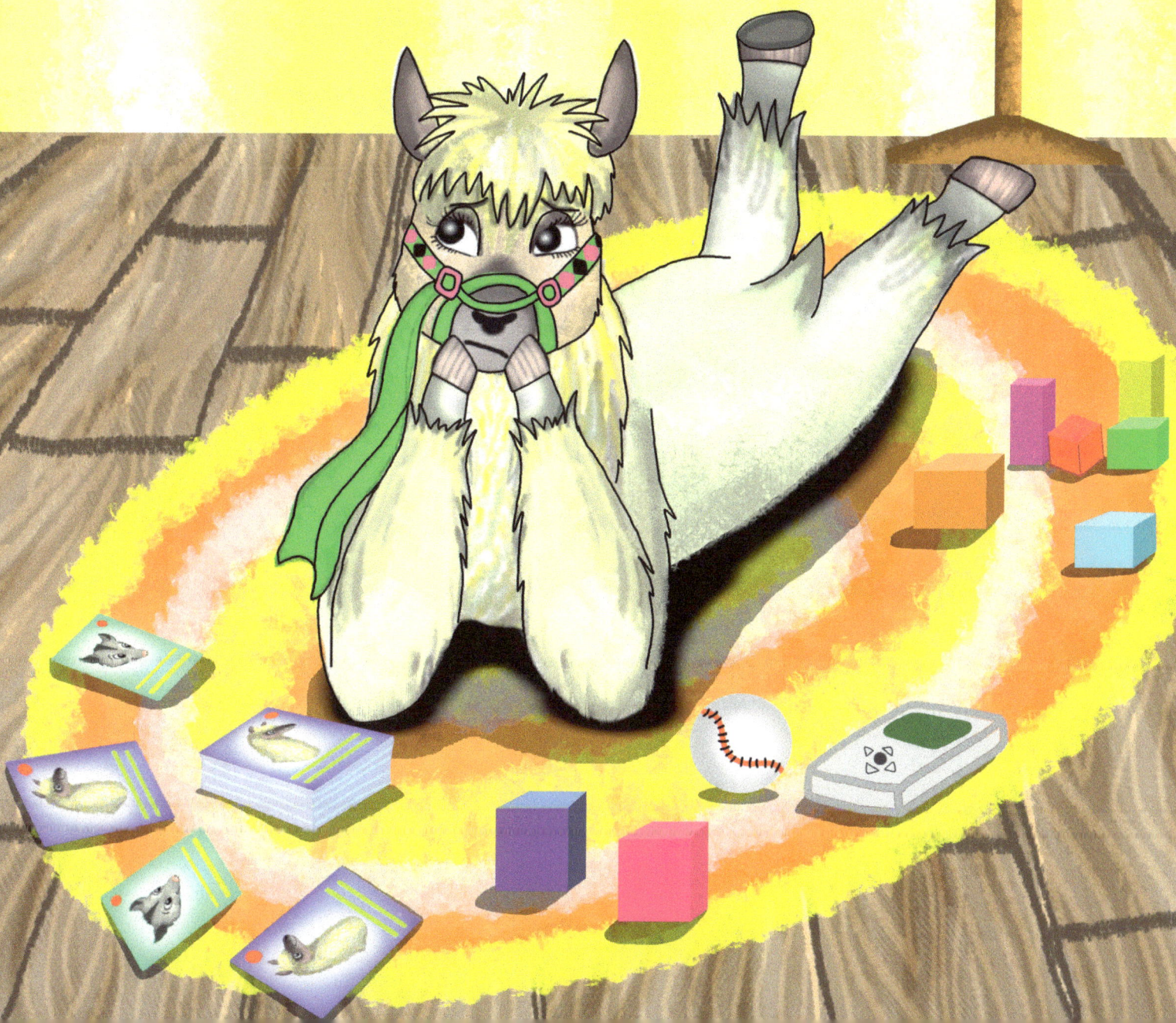

I rode my bike with Llama Stan.
"Stan, this biking is a great brain plan."

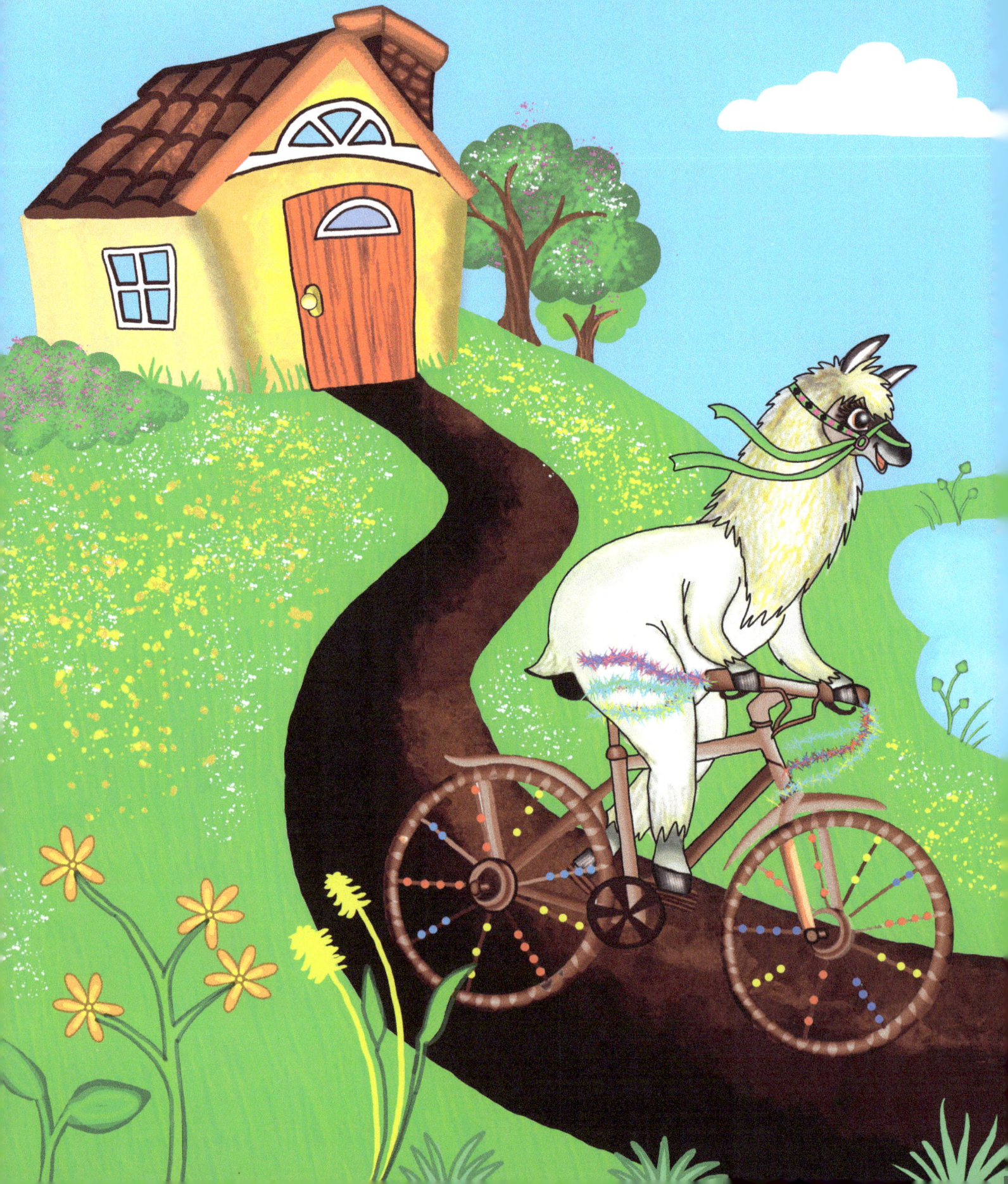

"My calm thoughts aren't hocus-pocus.
Biking gives me llama focus."

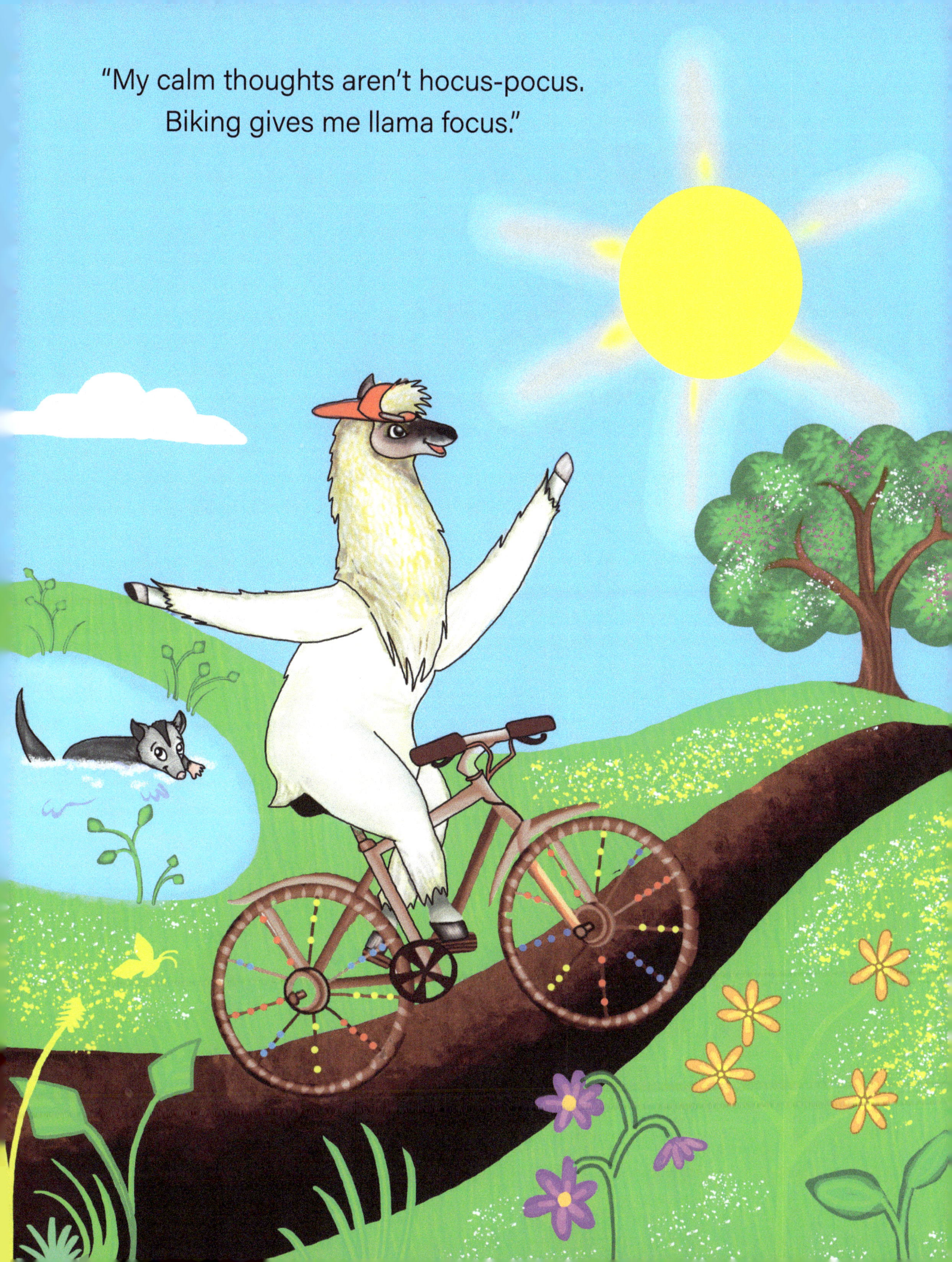

Llama locomotion is a super brain potion.

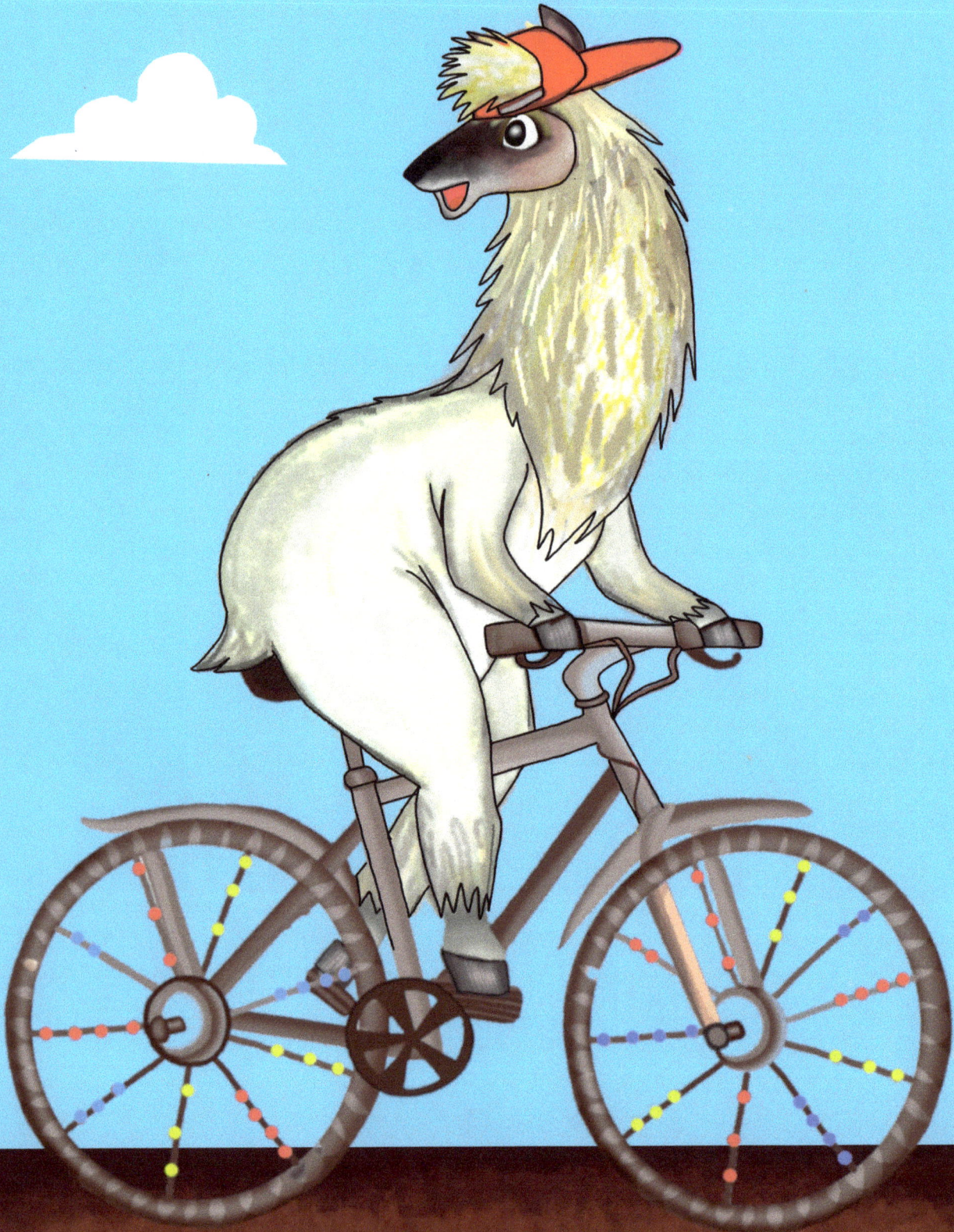

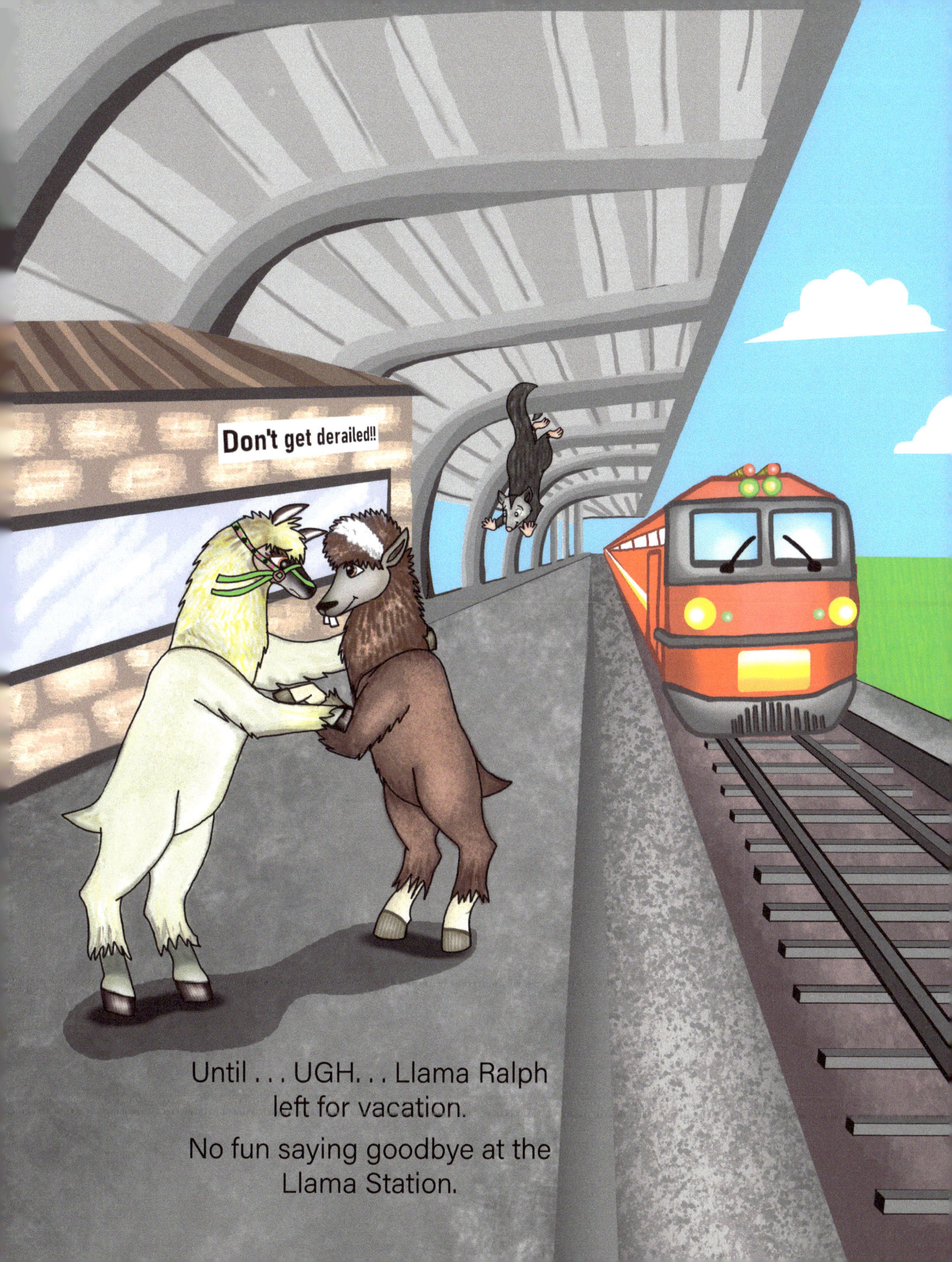

Don't get derailed!!

Until . . . UGH. . . Llama Ralph
left for vacation.
No fun saying goodbye at the
Llama Station.

"My body feels sluggish and very still.
I feel like I pushed Henry Goat straight uphill."

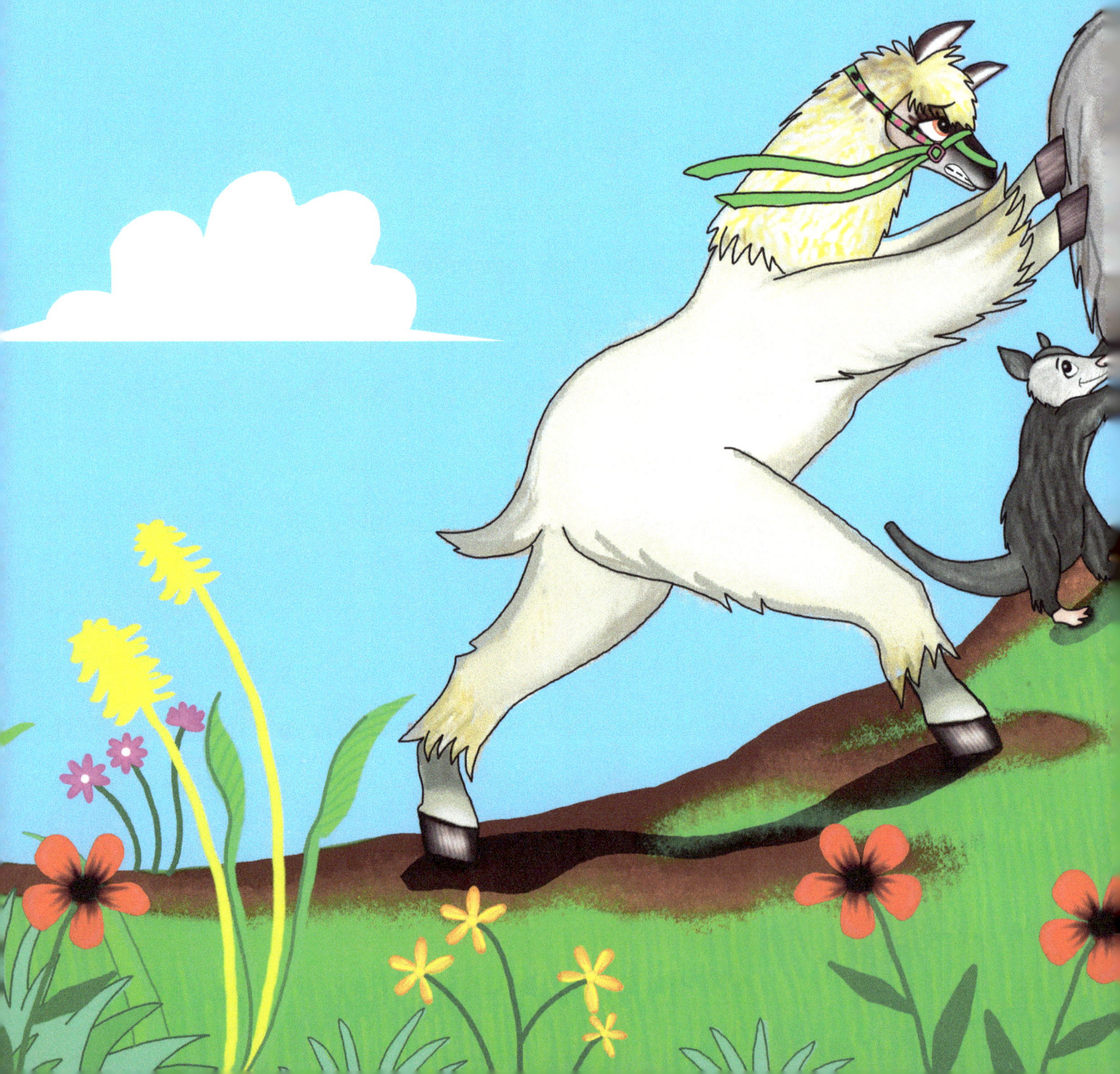

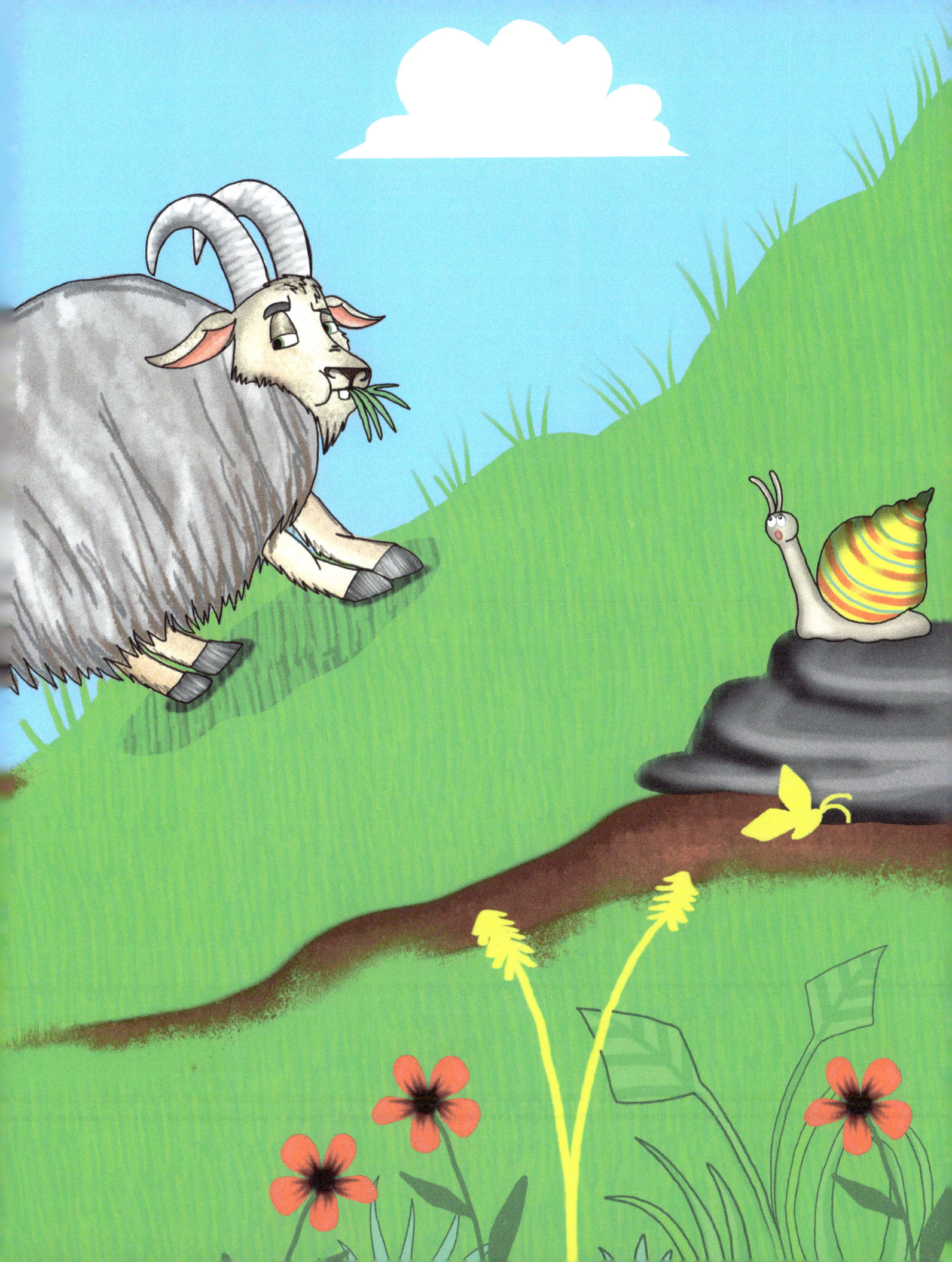

"Sammy," Mamma Llama said, "I know you feel sad to see Ralph go.
Be kind to yourself, and you may find low moods will come and go."

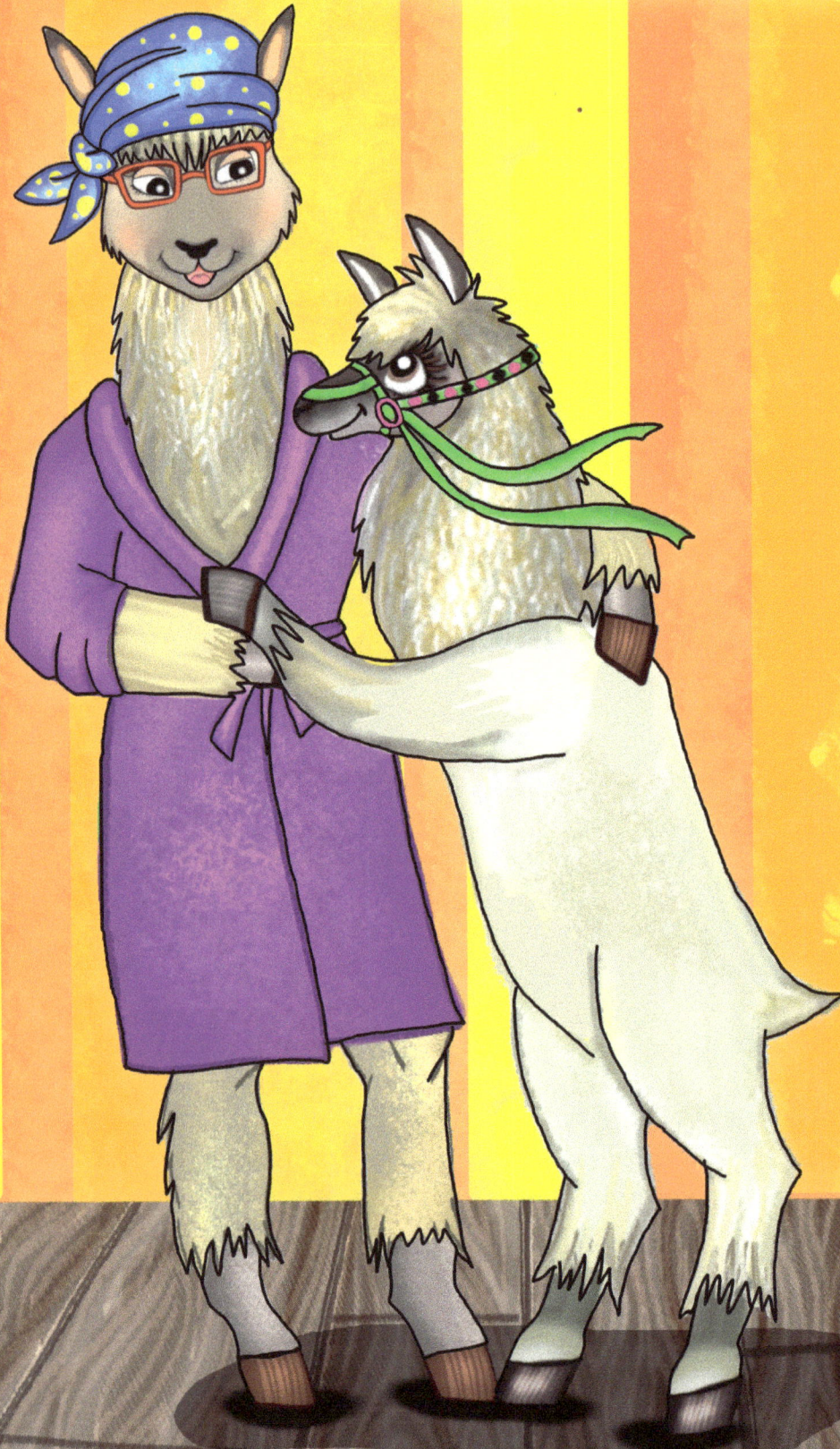

"Move your body and do something you like."

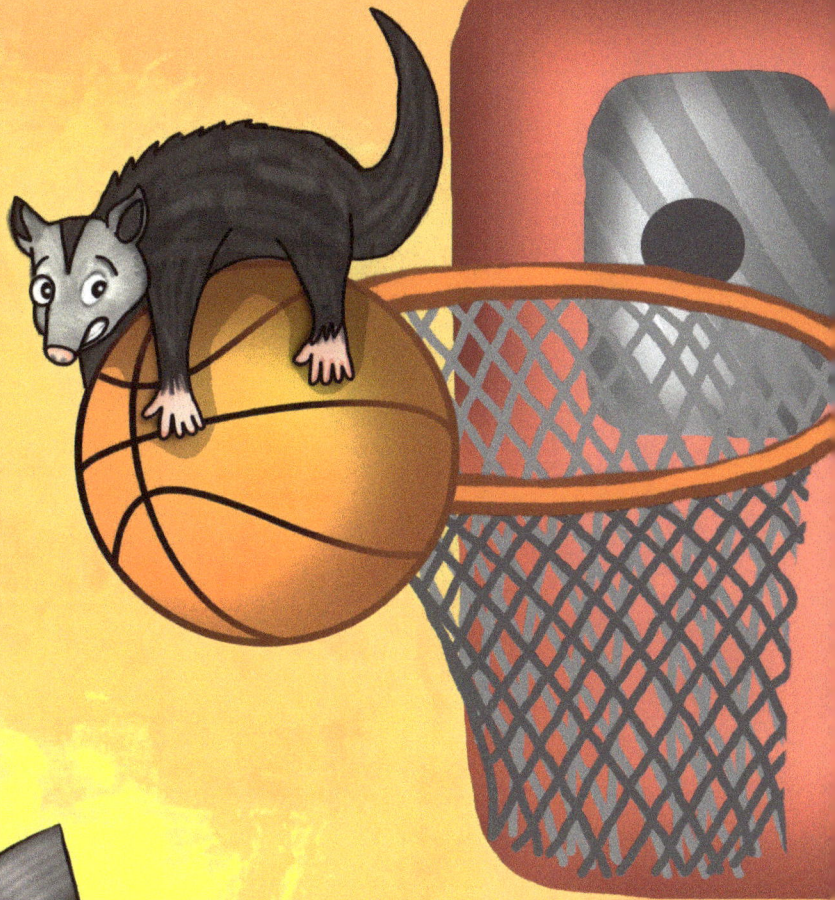

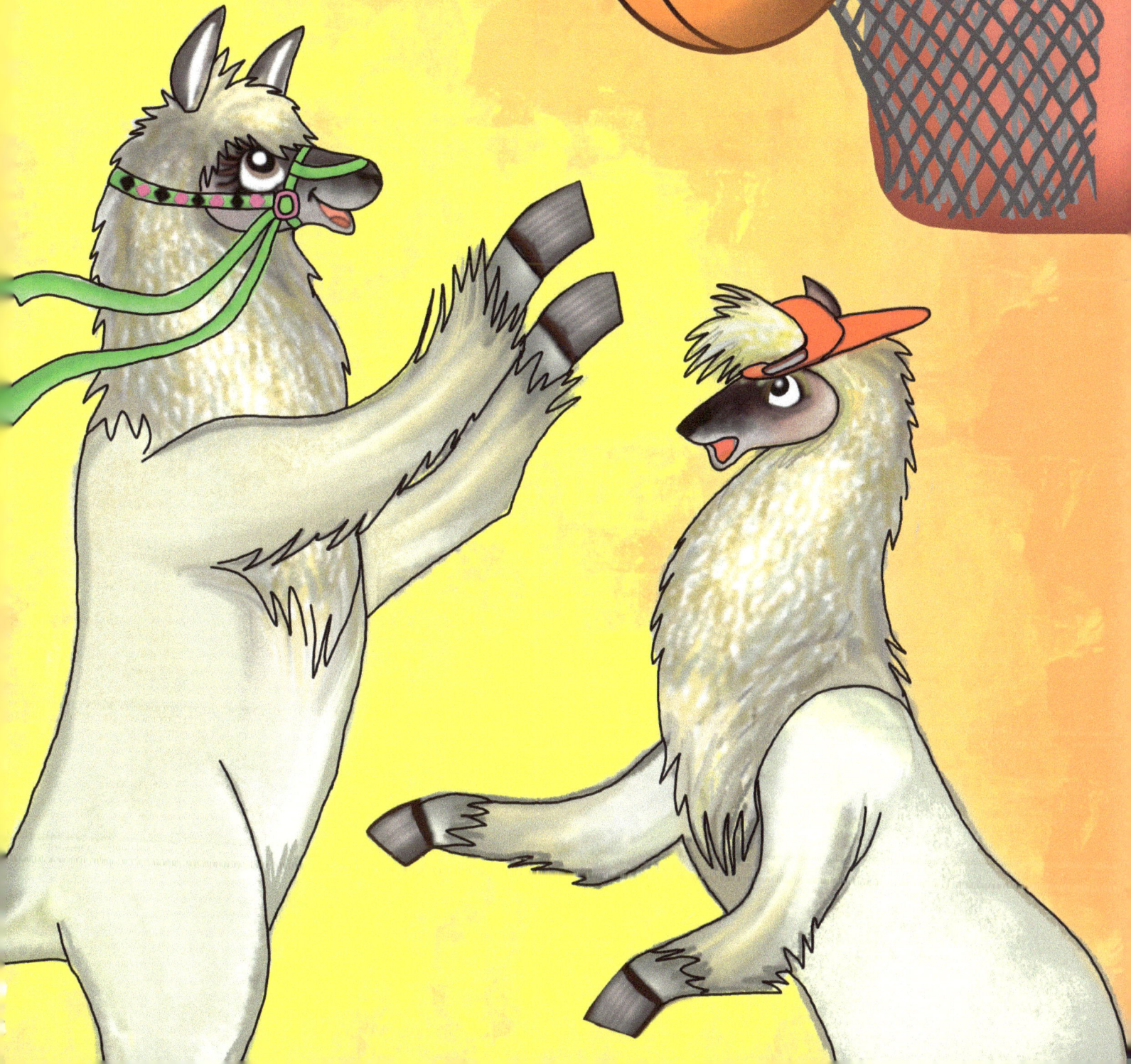

"You'll figure it out. Your body is wise."

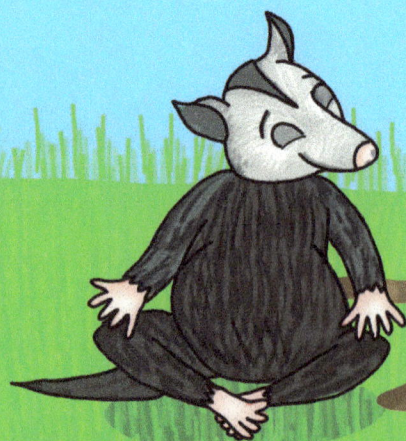

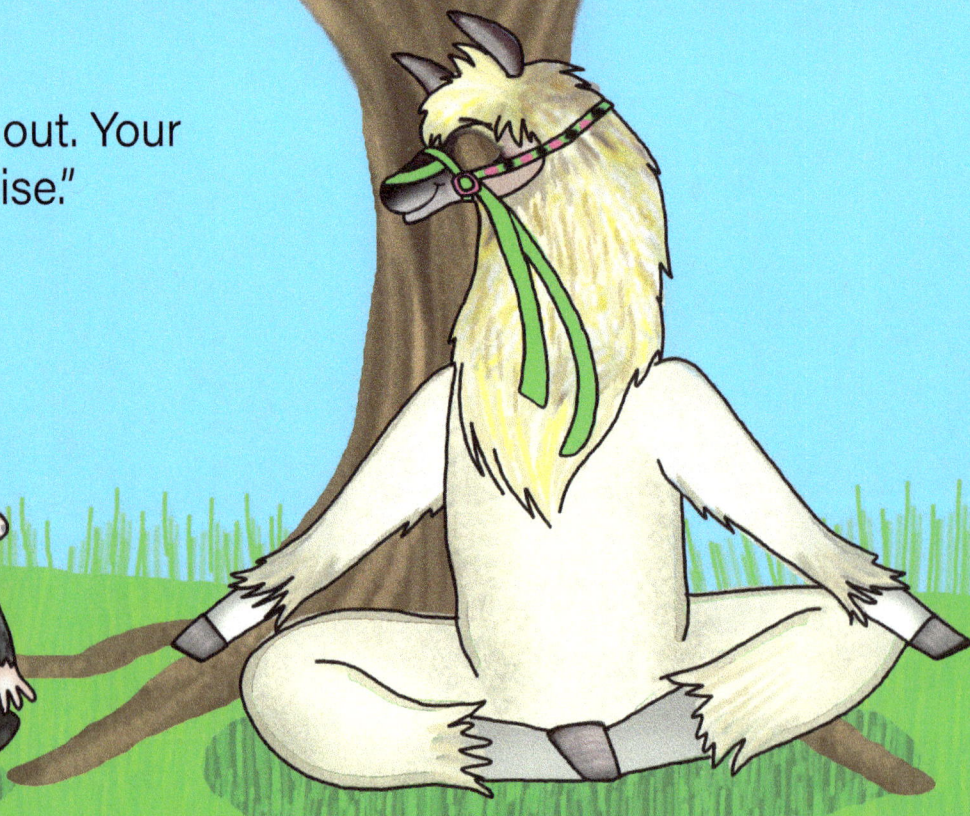

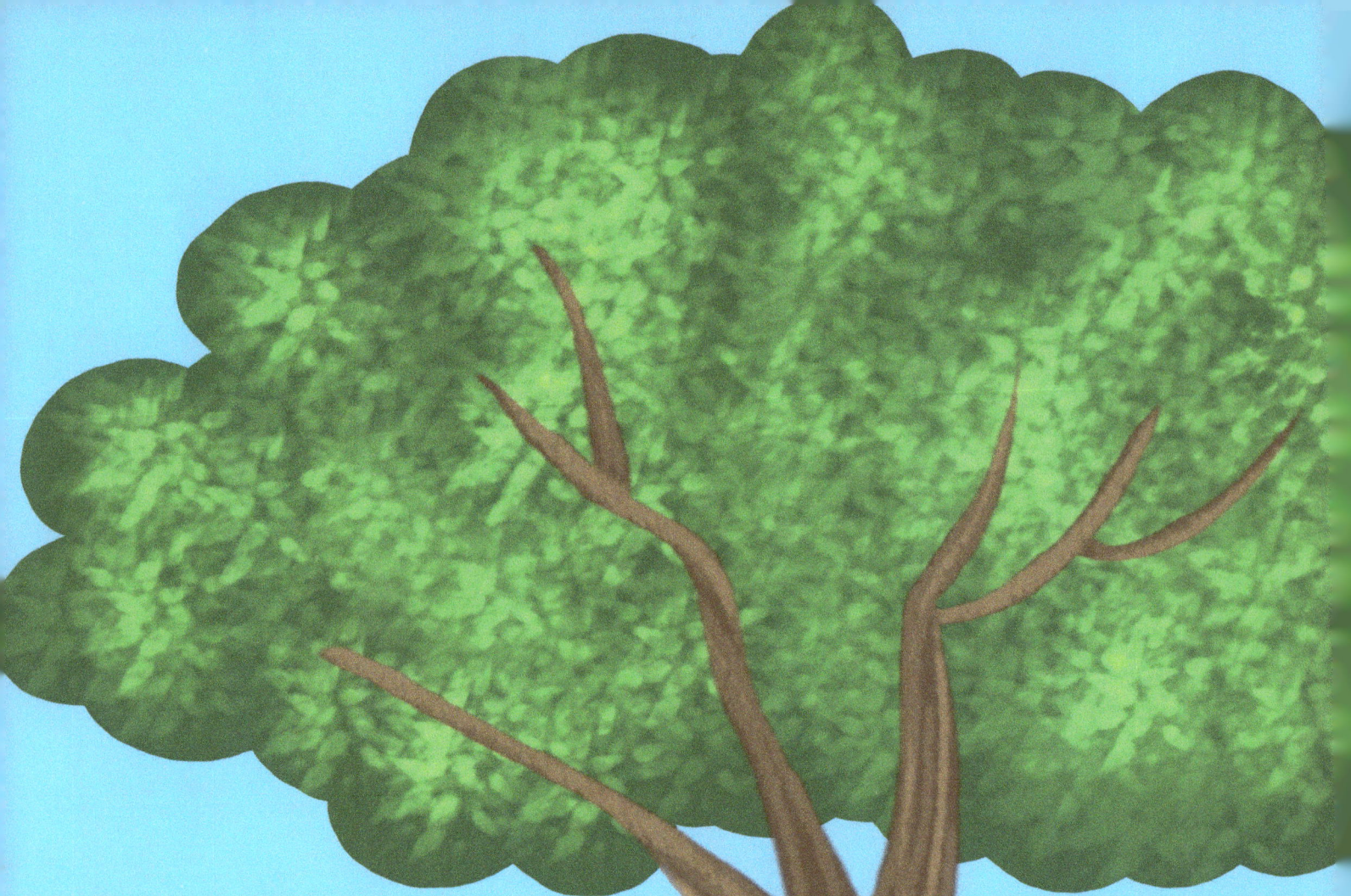

"Llamas often know just when to sit and when to rise."

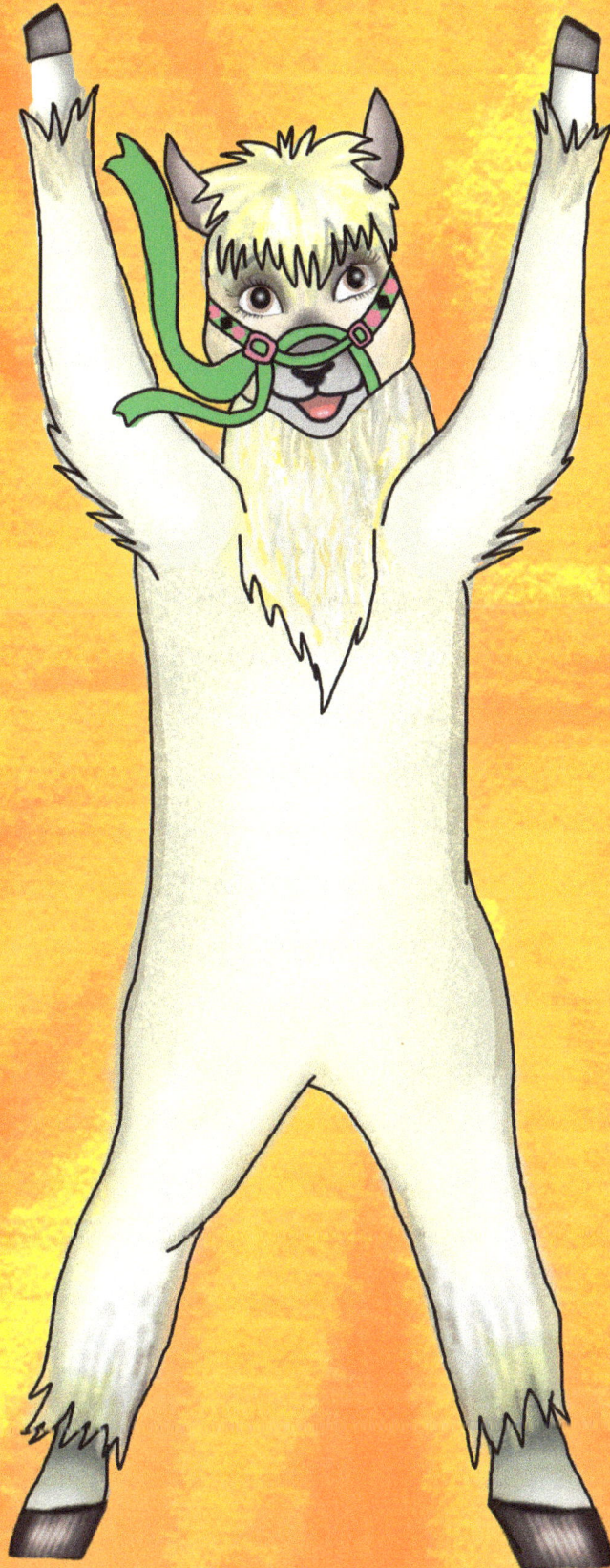

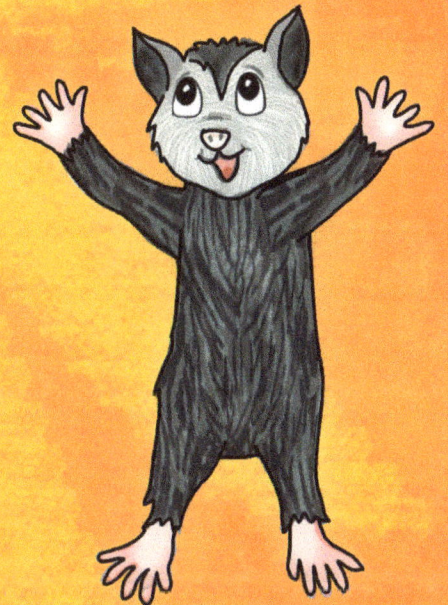

I looked up and down my whole city block.

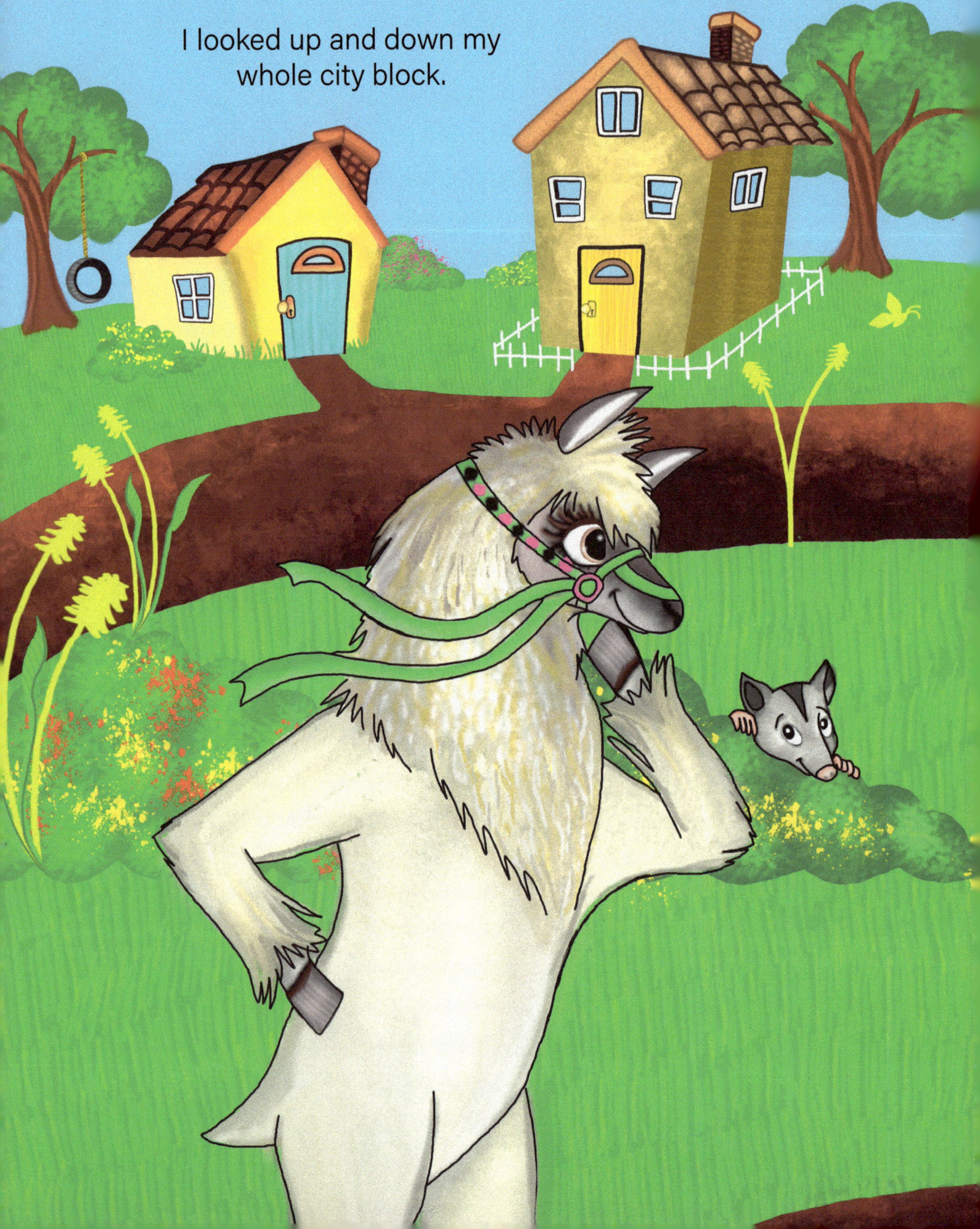

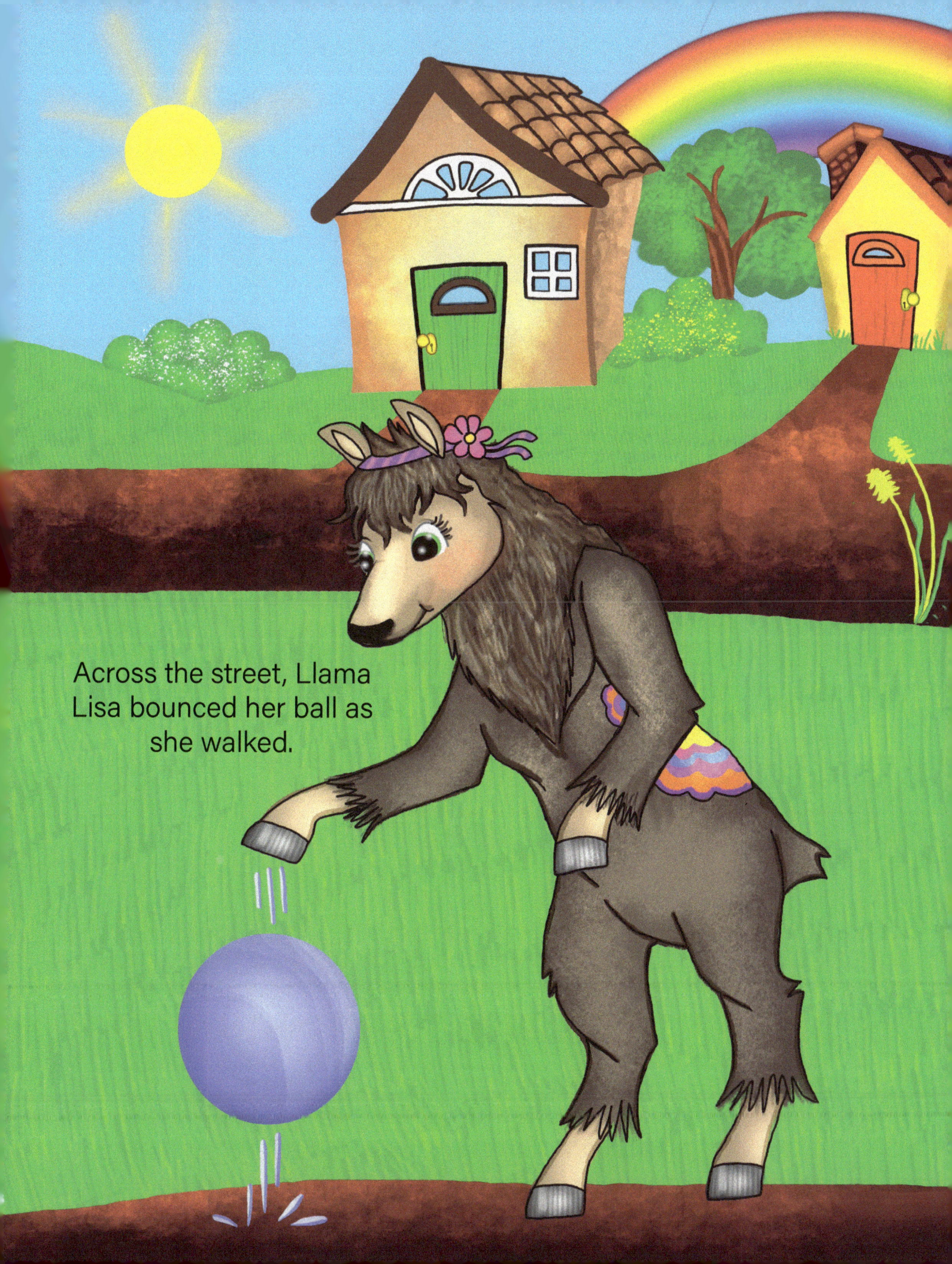

Across the street, Llama Lisa bounced her ball as she walked.

I drew 2-square boxes on the sidewalk with
my bright blue llama chalk.
"Lisa, let's play 2-square."

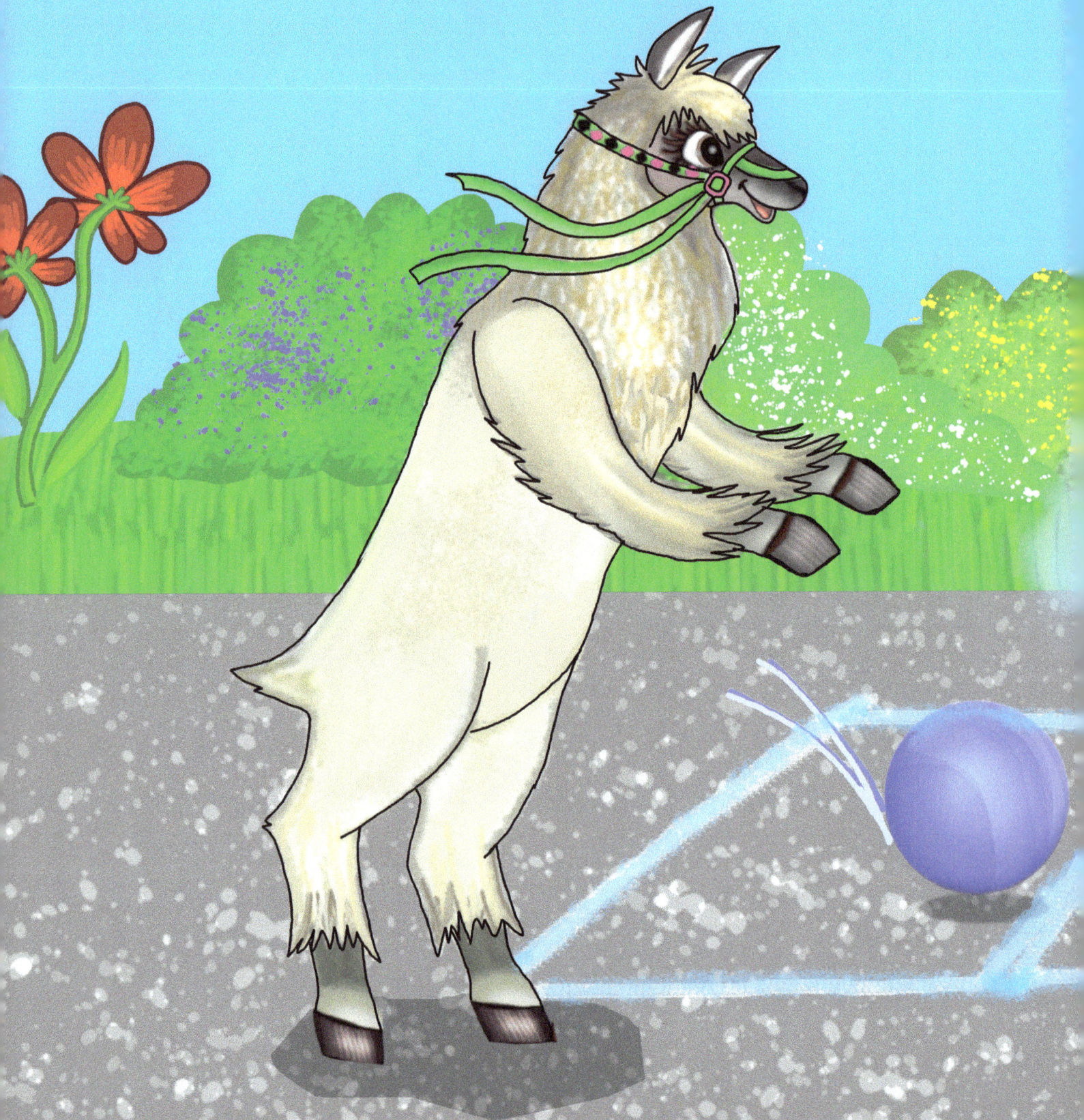

Lisa laughed, "This is a blast."

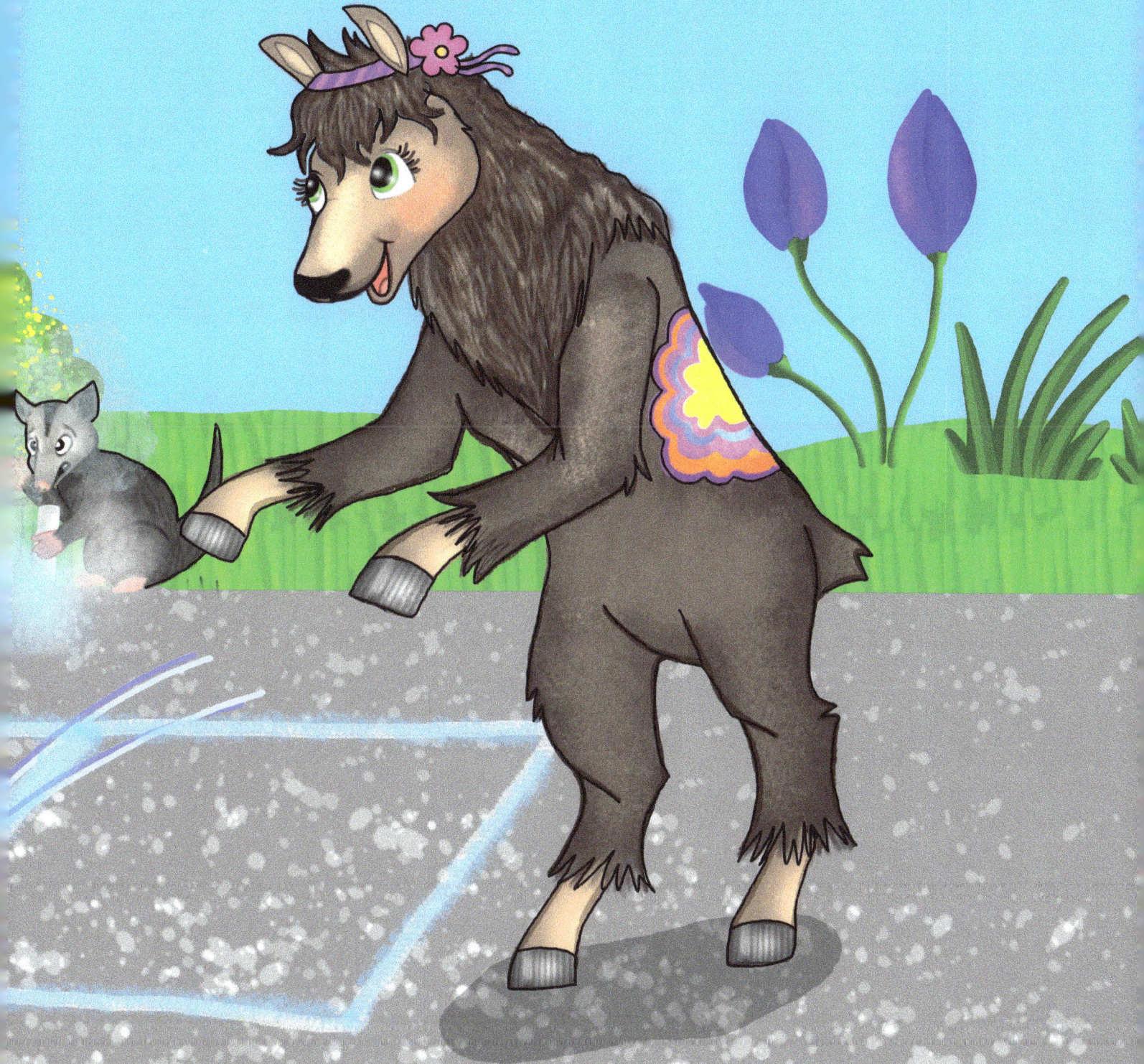

Bouncing is a fun llama motion.
Bouncing boosted happy potion.

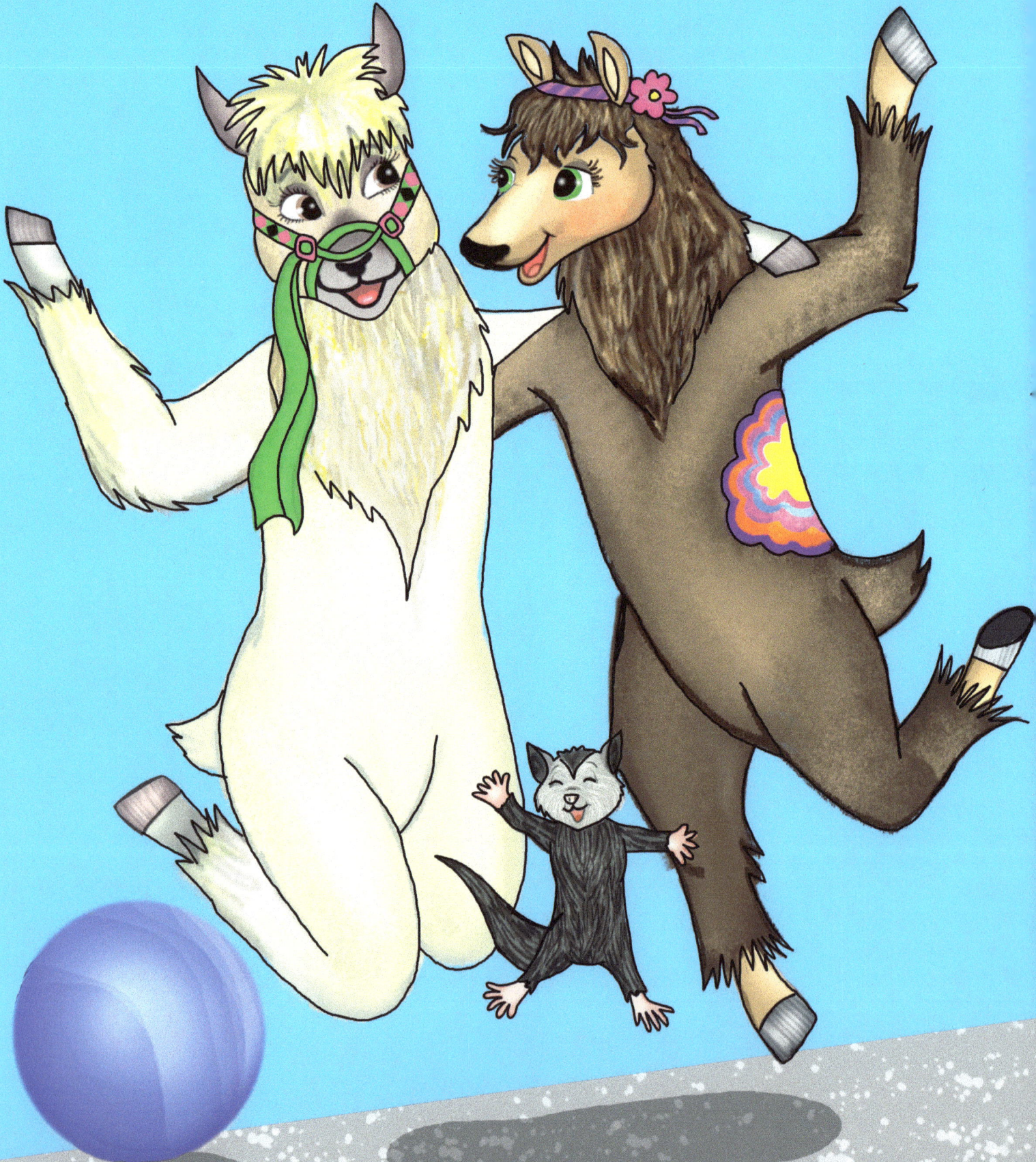

Until . . . UGH . . . I'll tell you what happened in school today.

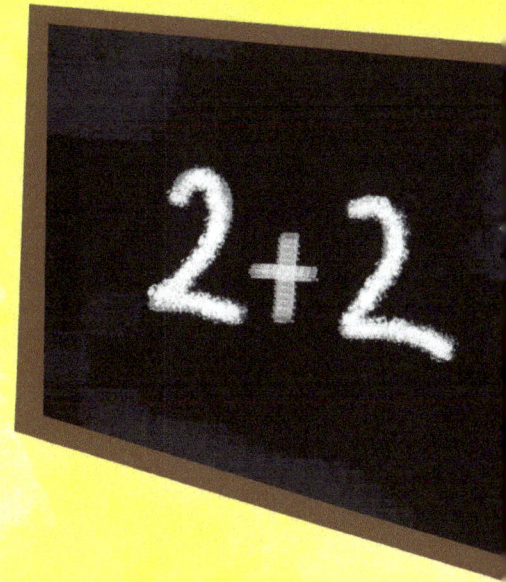

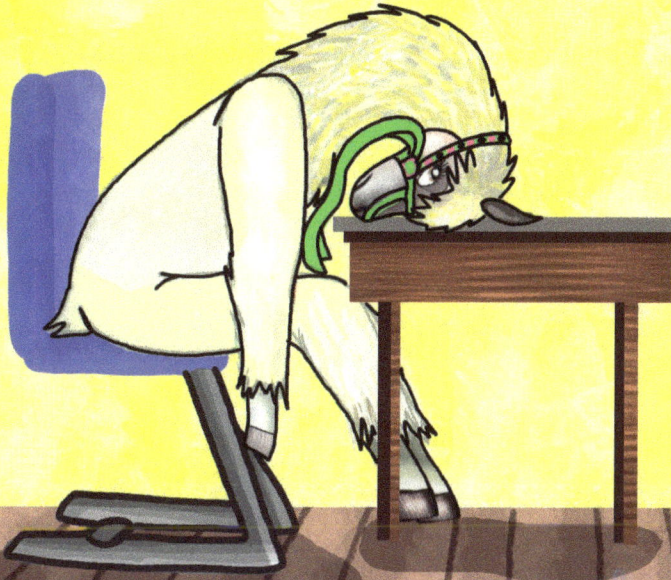

2+2

I felt zero happy potion.
Sitting still is just not my way.

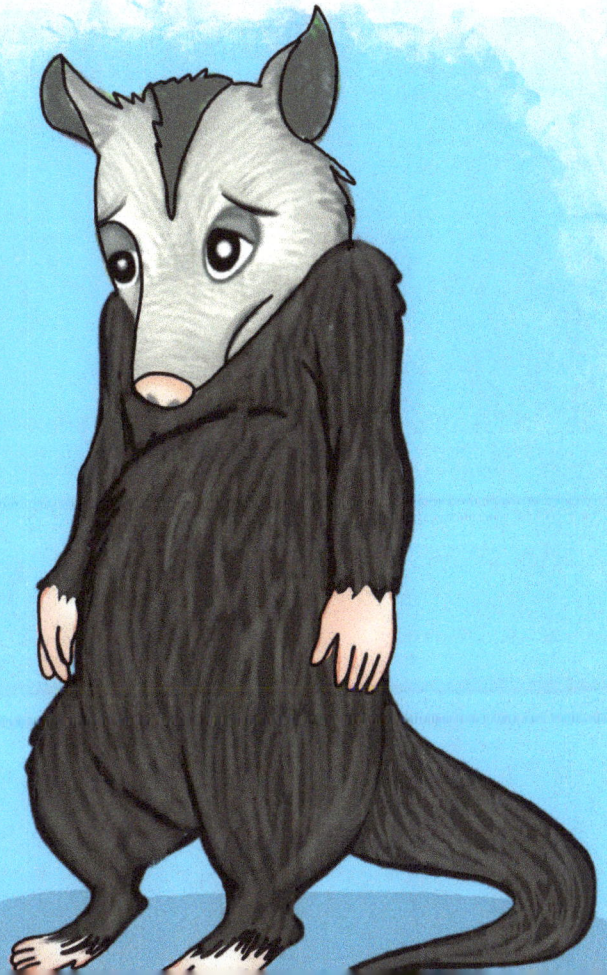

Mrs. Llama Phi called me to the chalkboard to
answer 2 + 2 in front of my whole class.
I asked if I could pass.
"My brain tank is empty," I shouted.

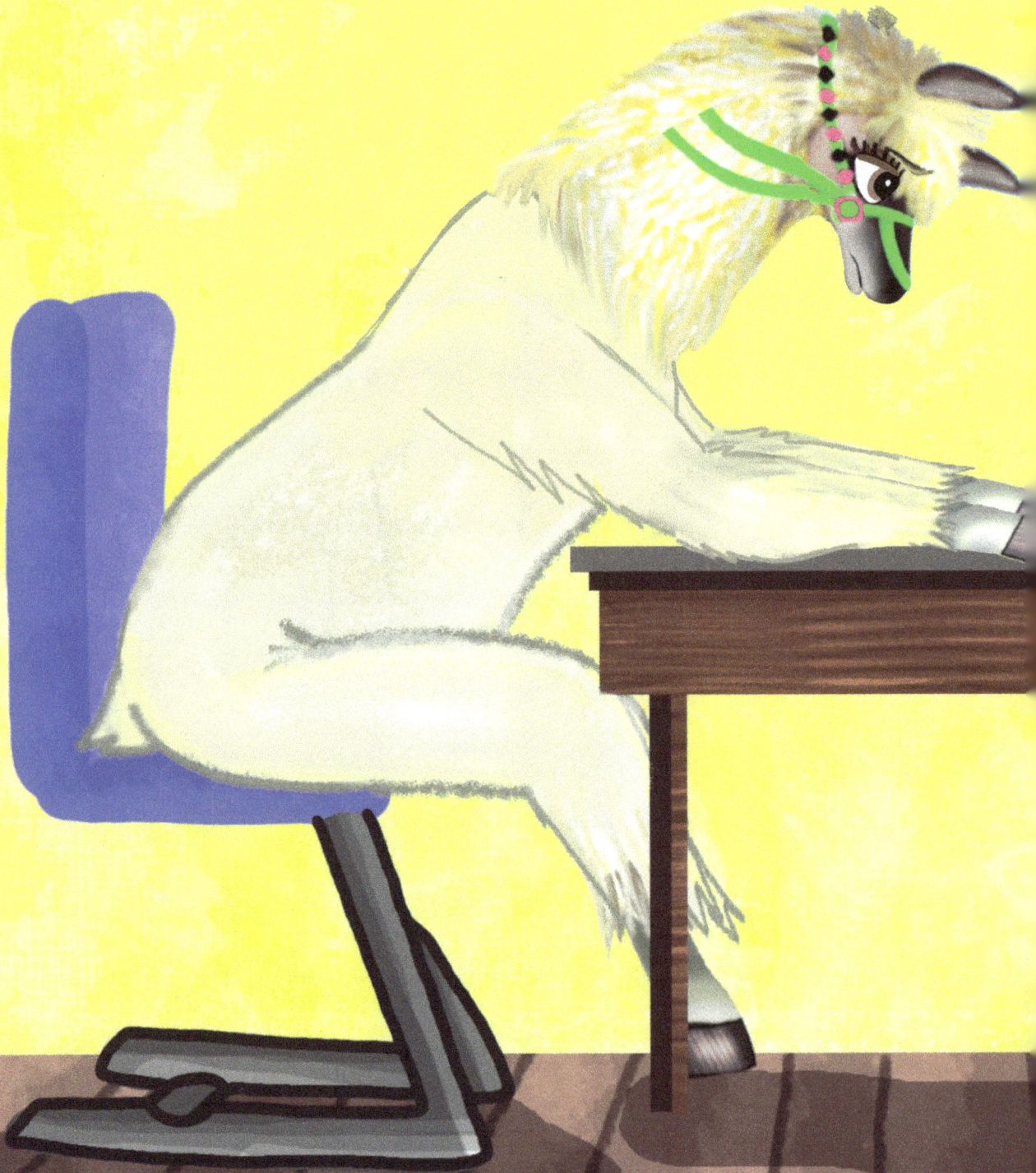

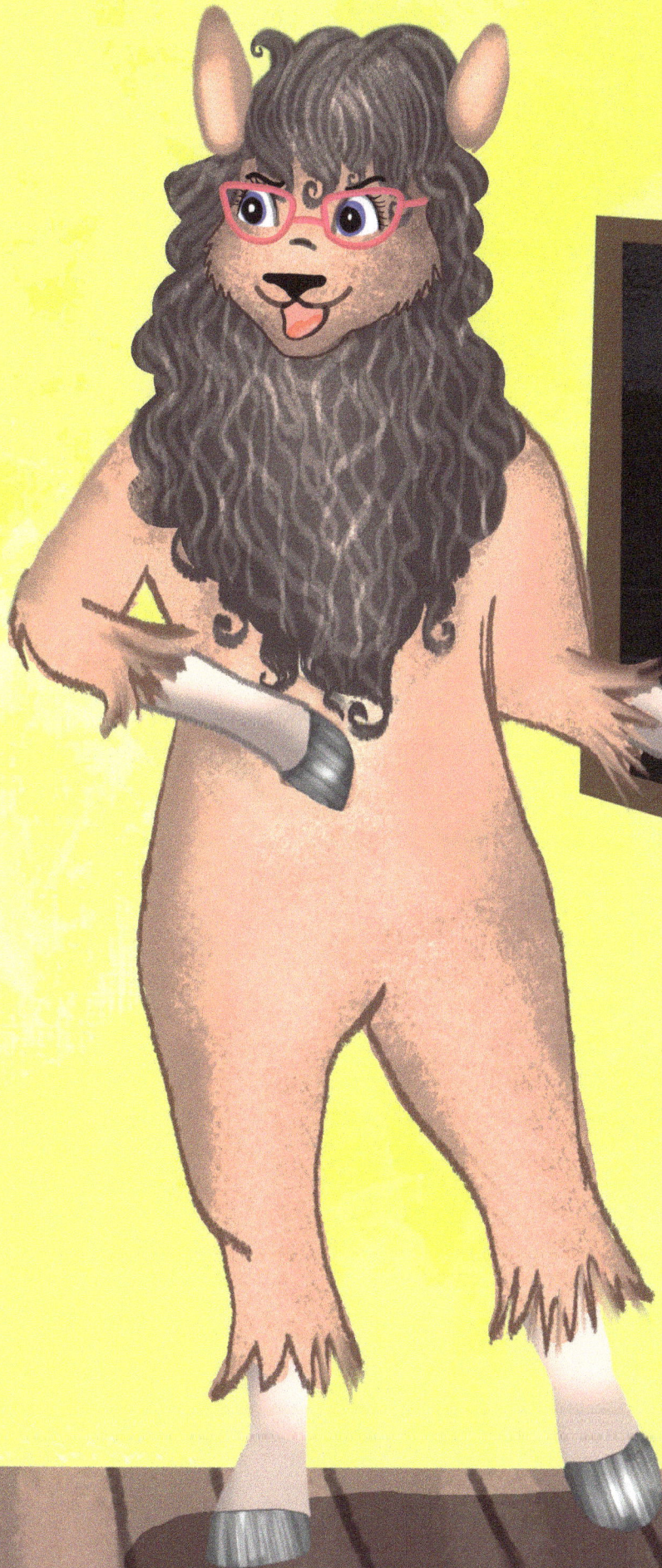

My shoulders slumped,
my mouth in a pout;
my still body was very
spaced out.

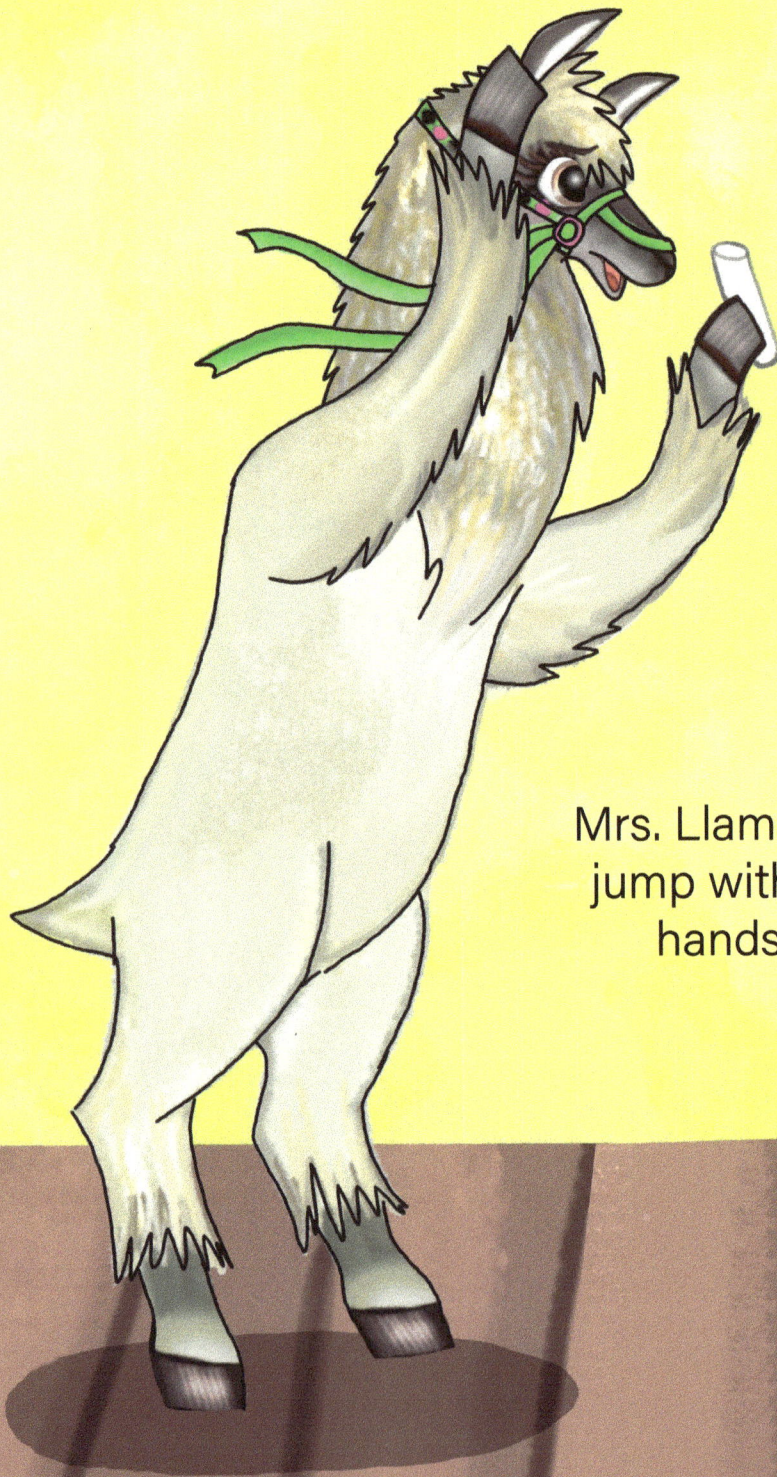

Mrs. Llama Phi said, "Let's jump with legs wide and hands to the side."

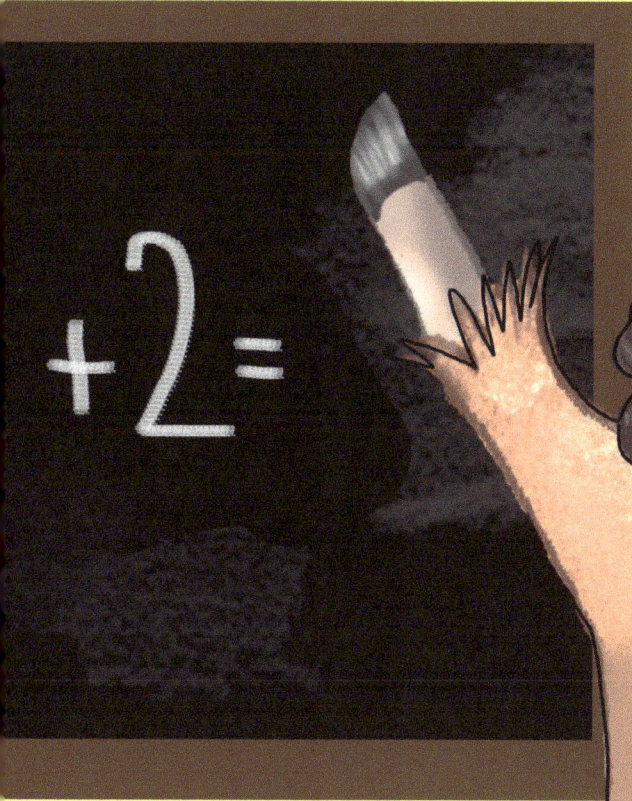

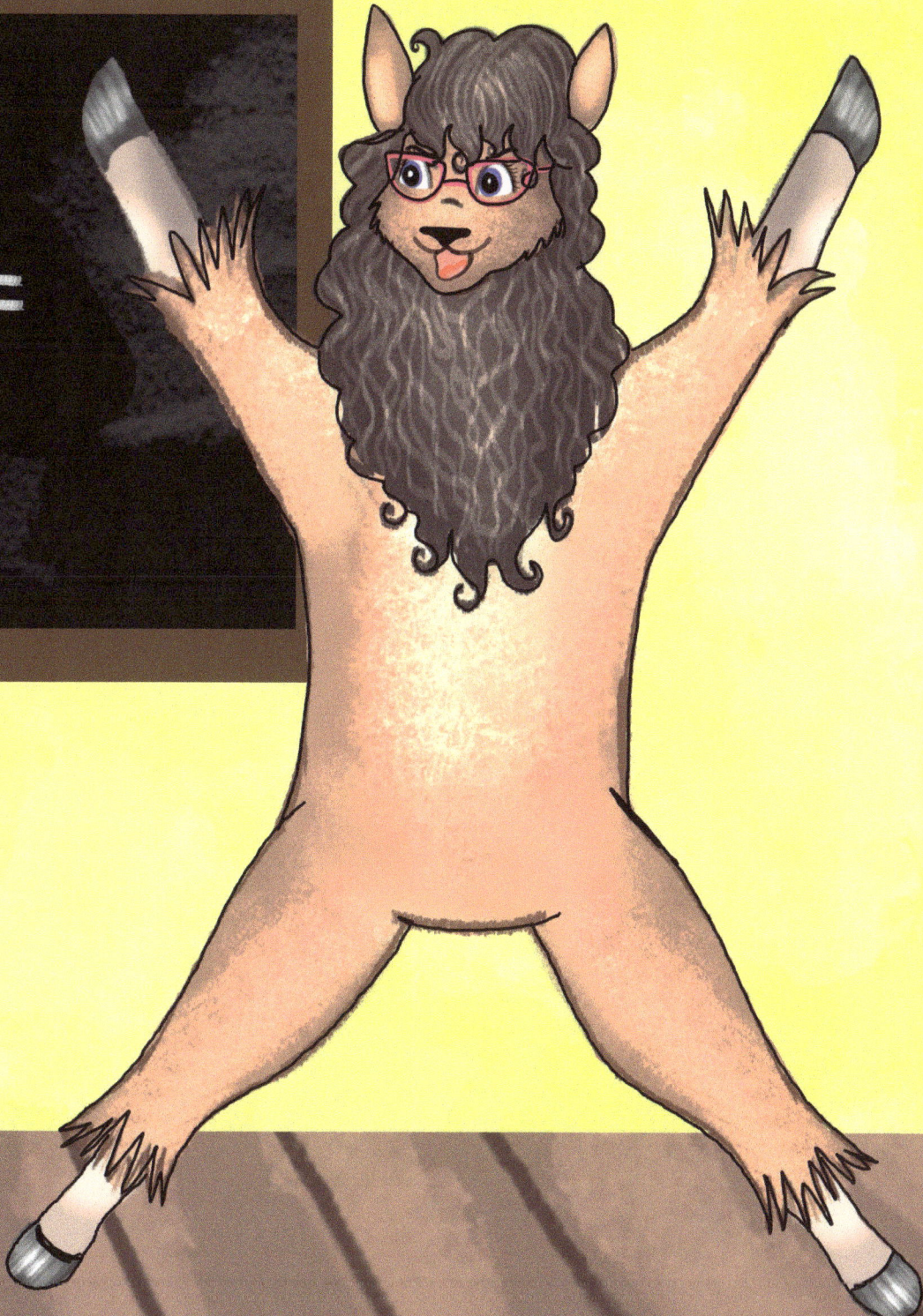

"Now, stand up and stretch and take a deep breath.
Do it again, and we'll begin."

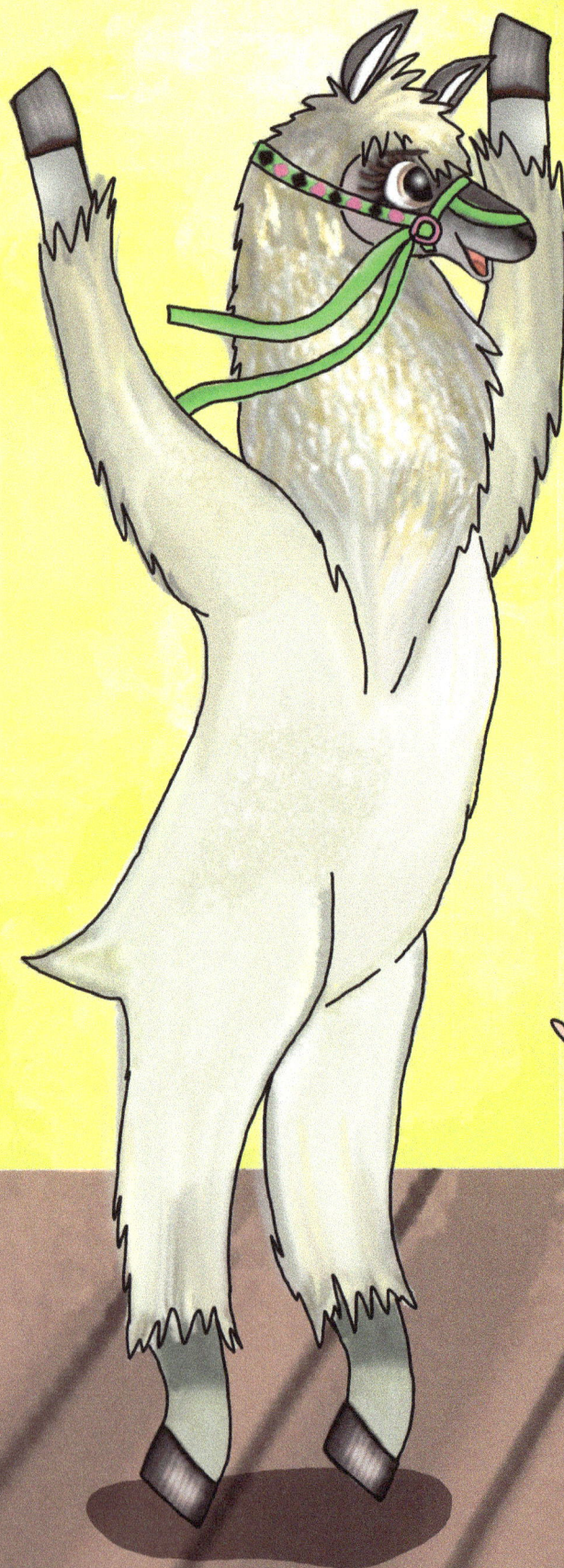

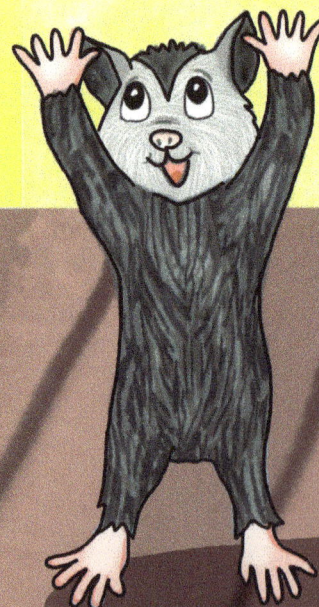

"Sammy, walk two of your classmates to the board. Count to two; now bring two more."

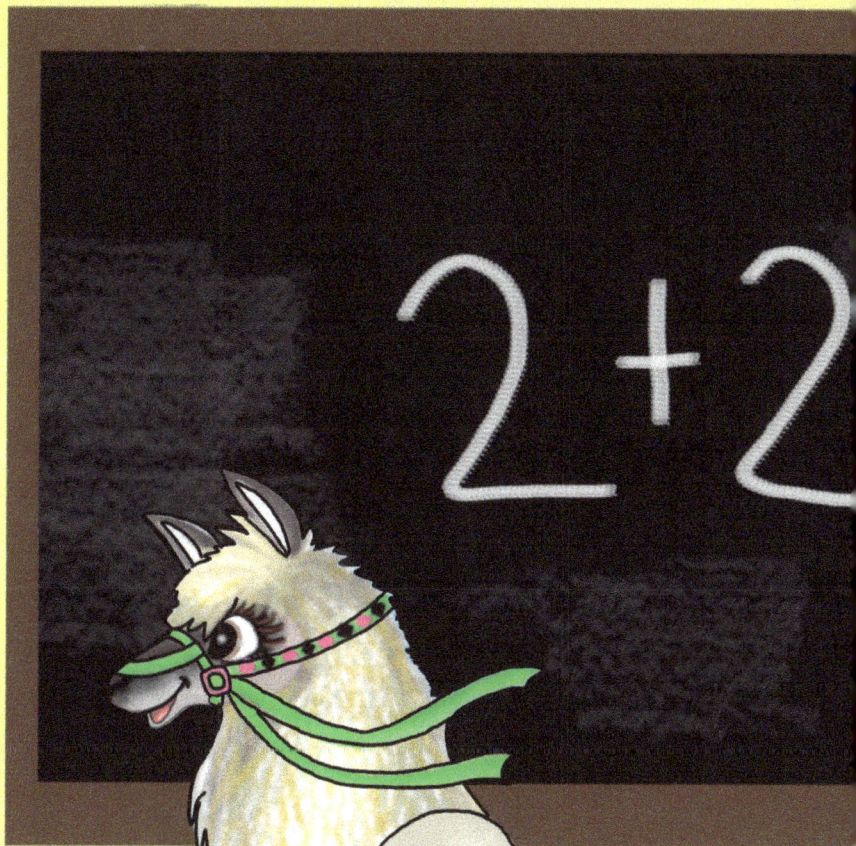

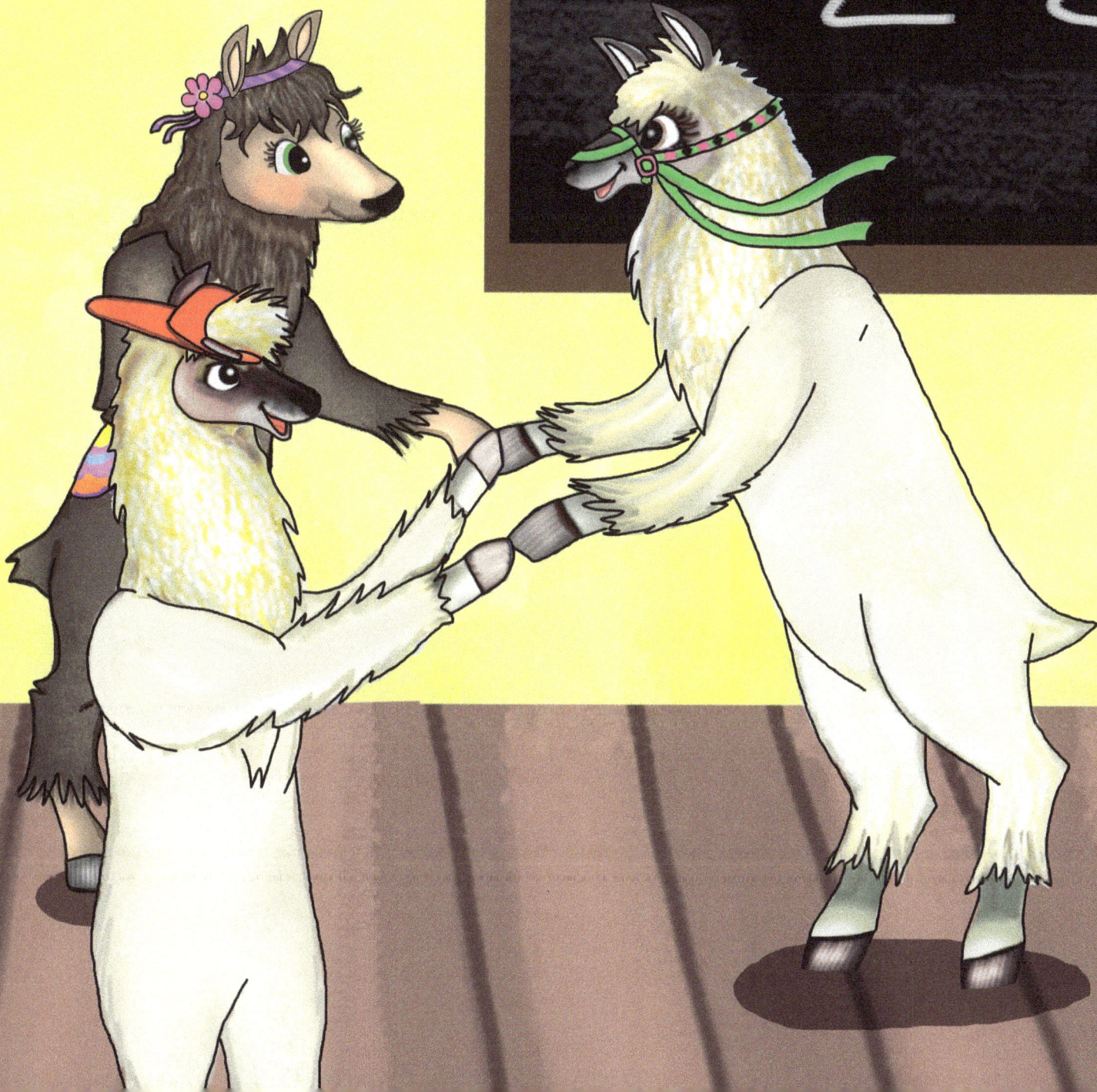

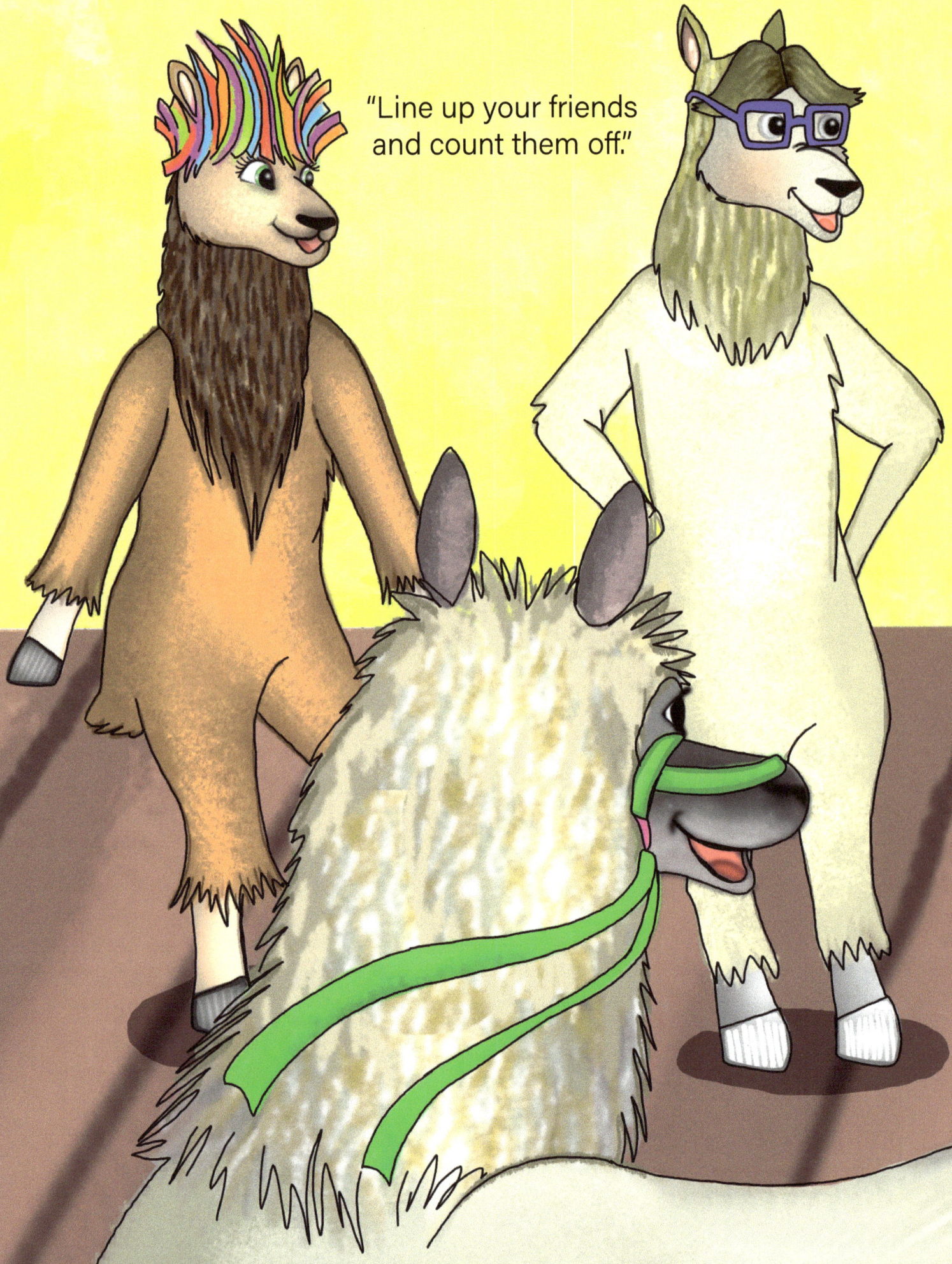

"Line up your friends and count them off."

I counted off one with Llama Laura...

And ended at four with Llama Cora.

The answer is FOUR! Let's celebrate!

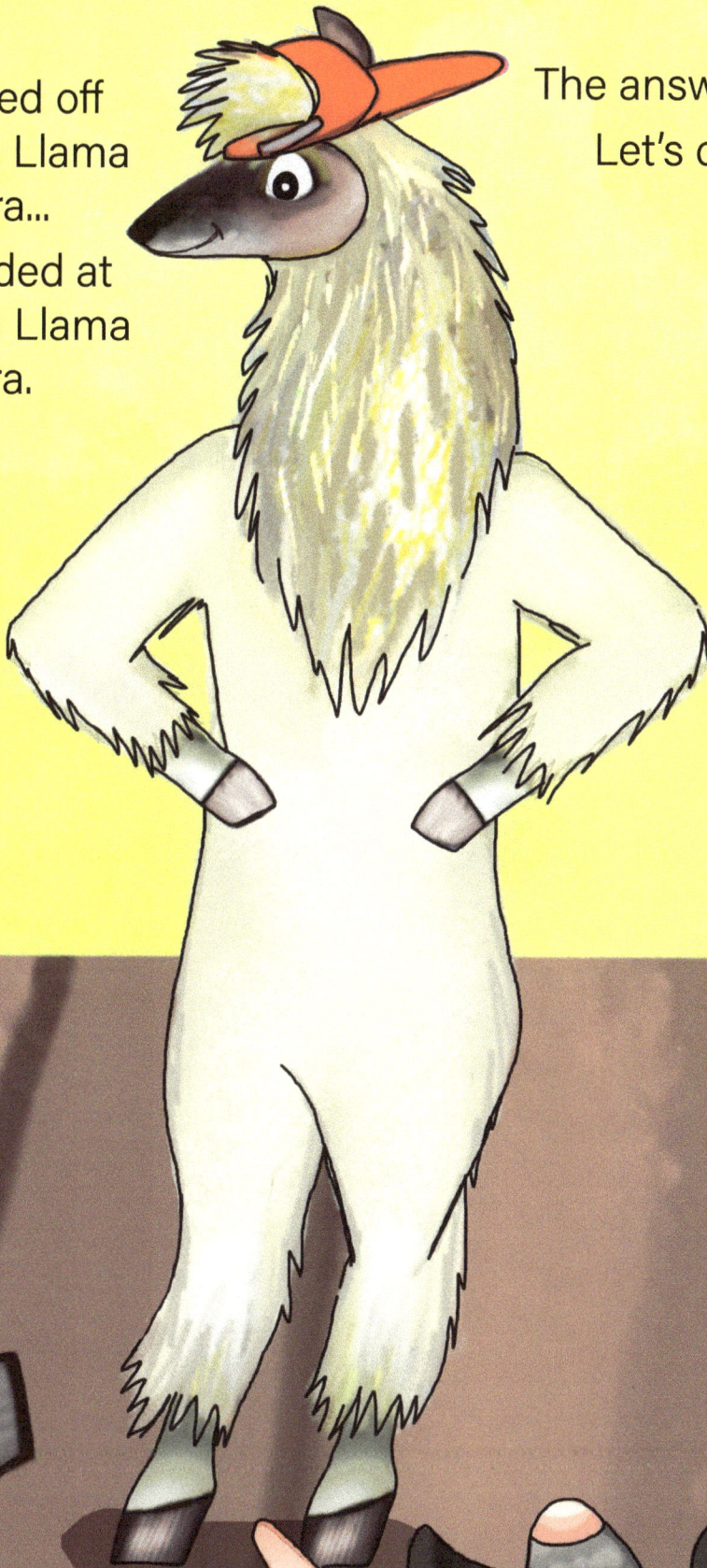

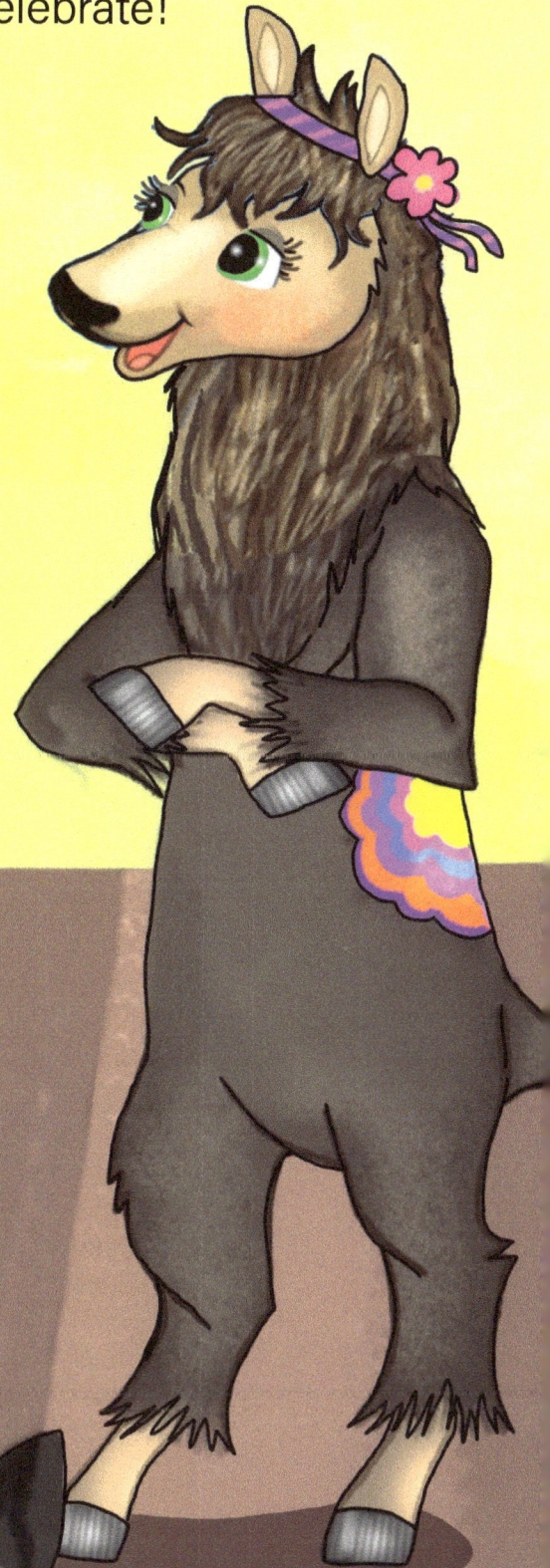

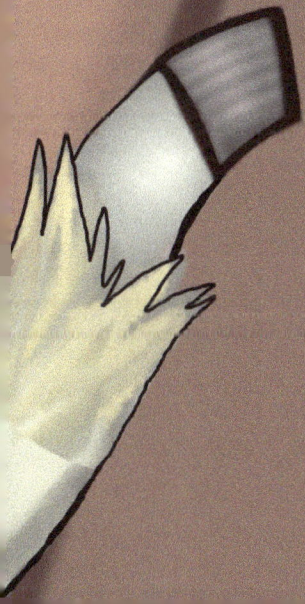

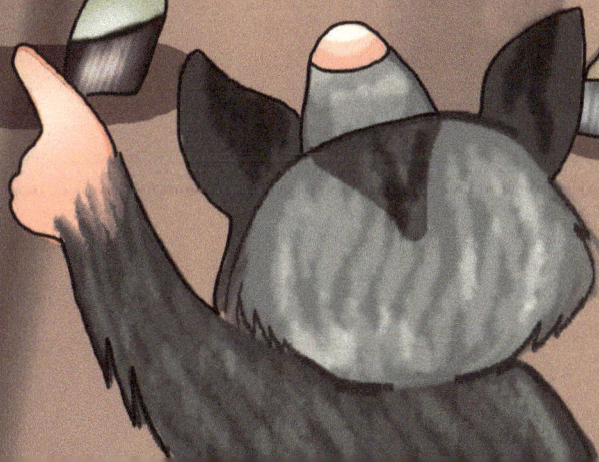

Llama locomotion is a smart brain potion.

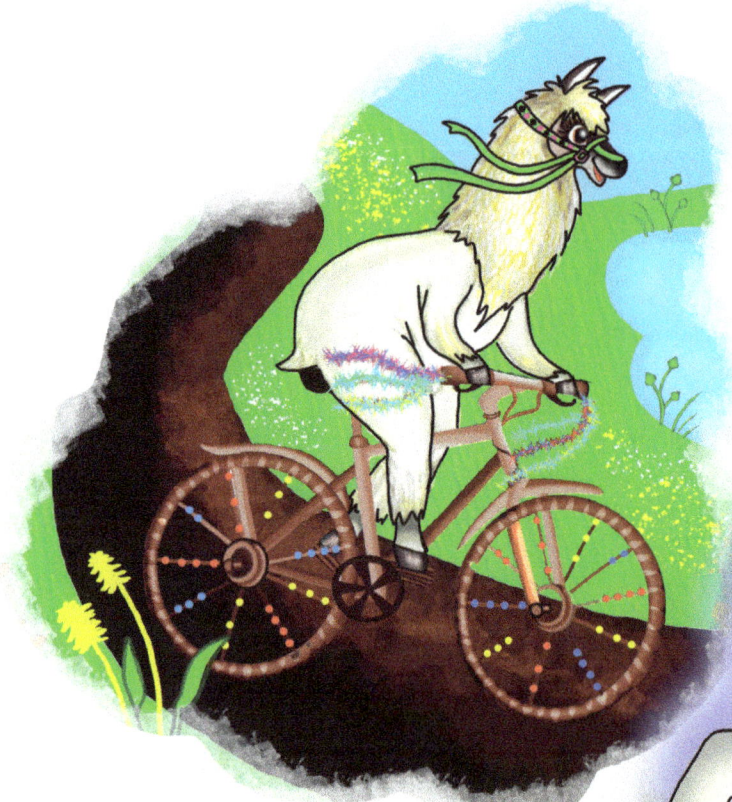

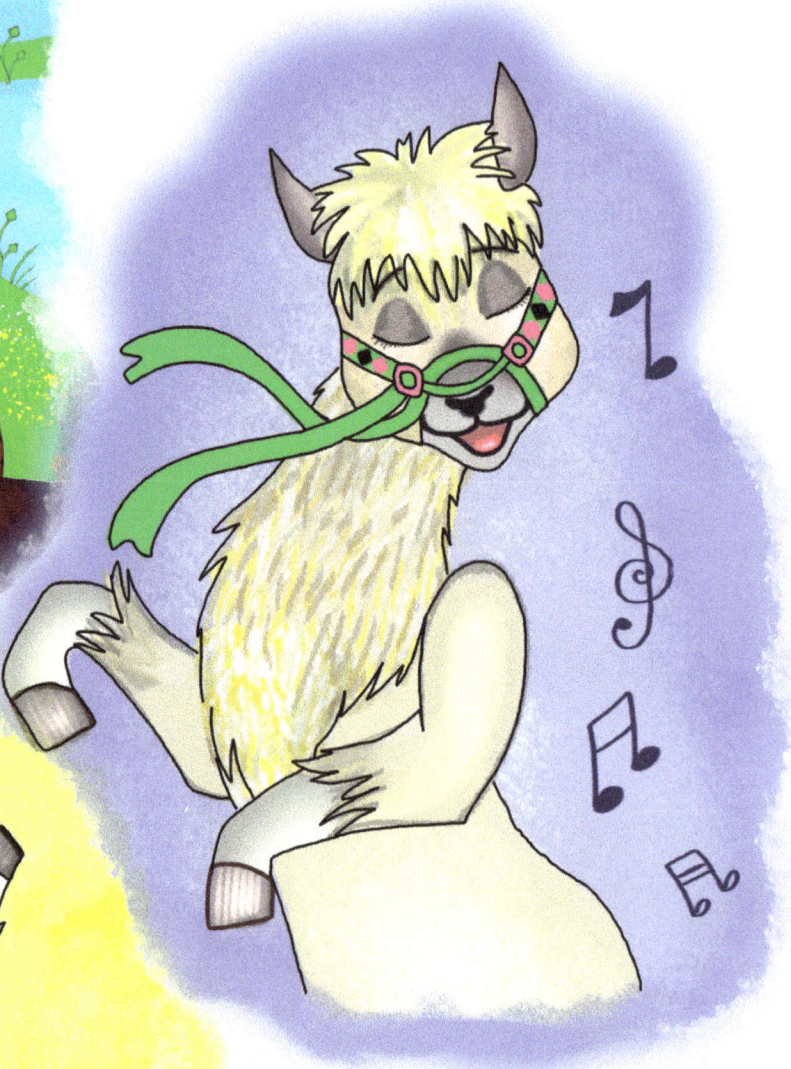

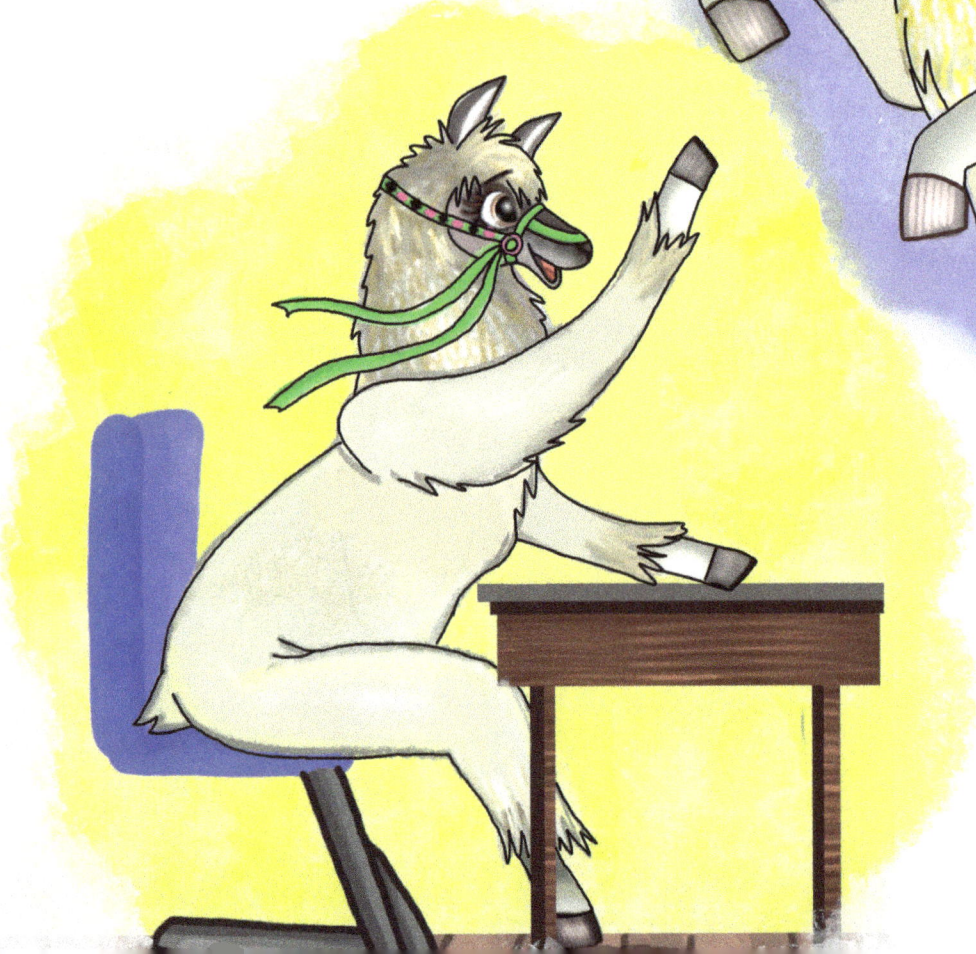

I honor my feelings with kindness and care.
My heart and my body are mindfully aware.

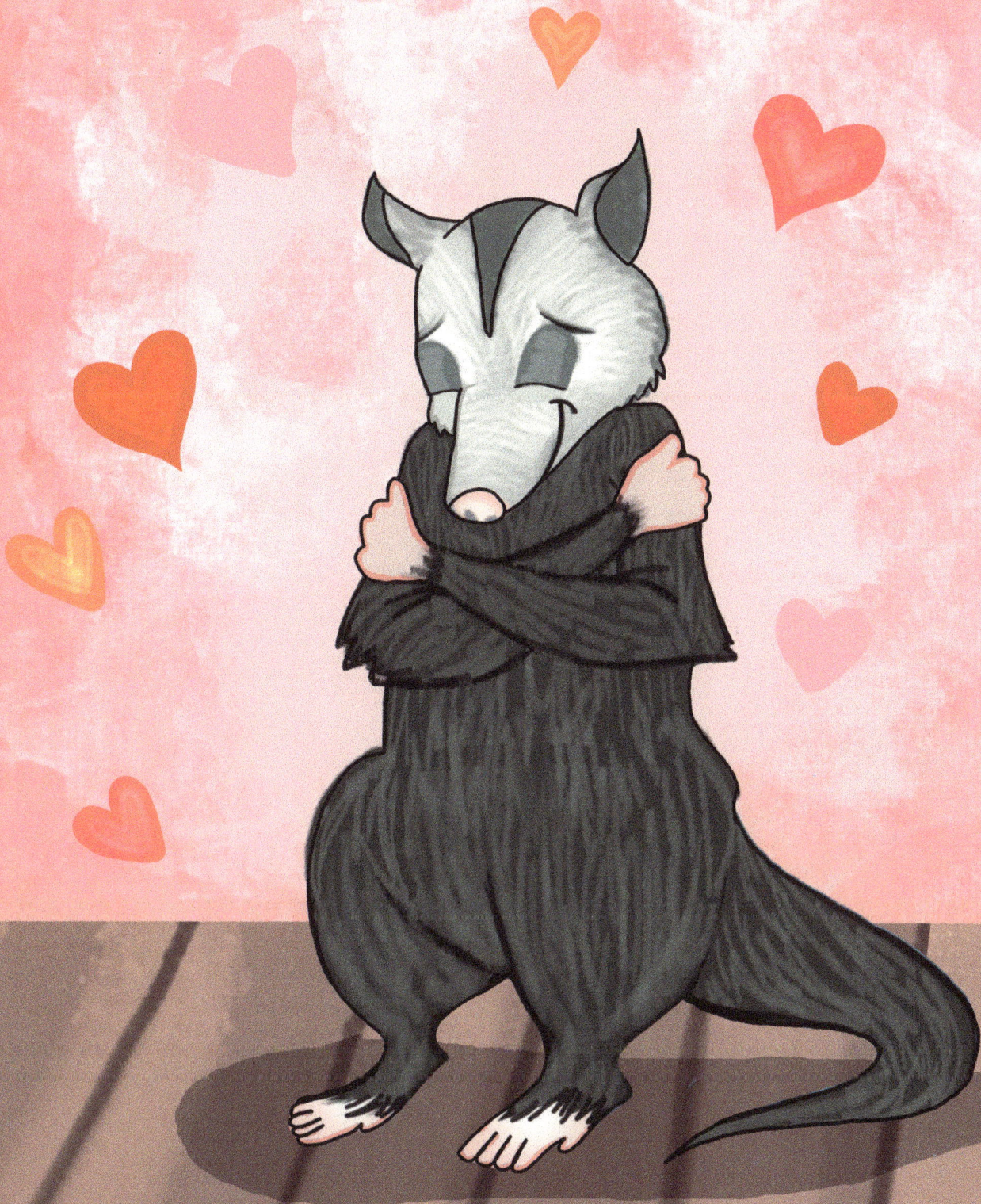

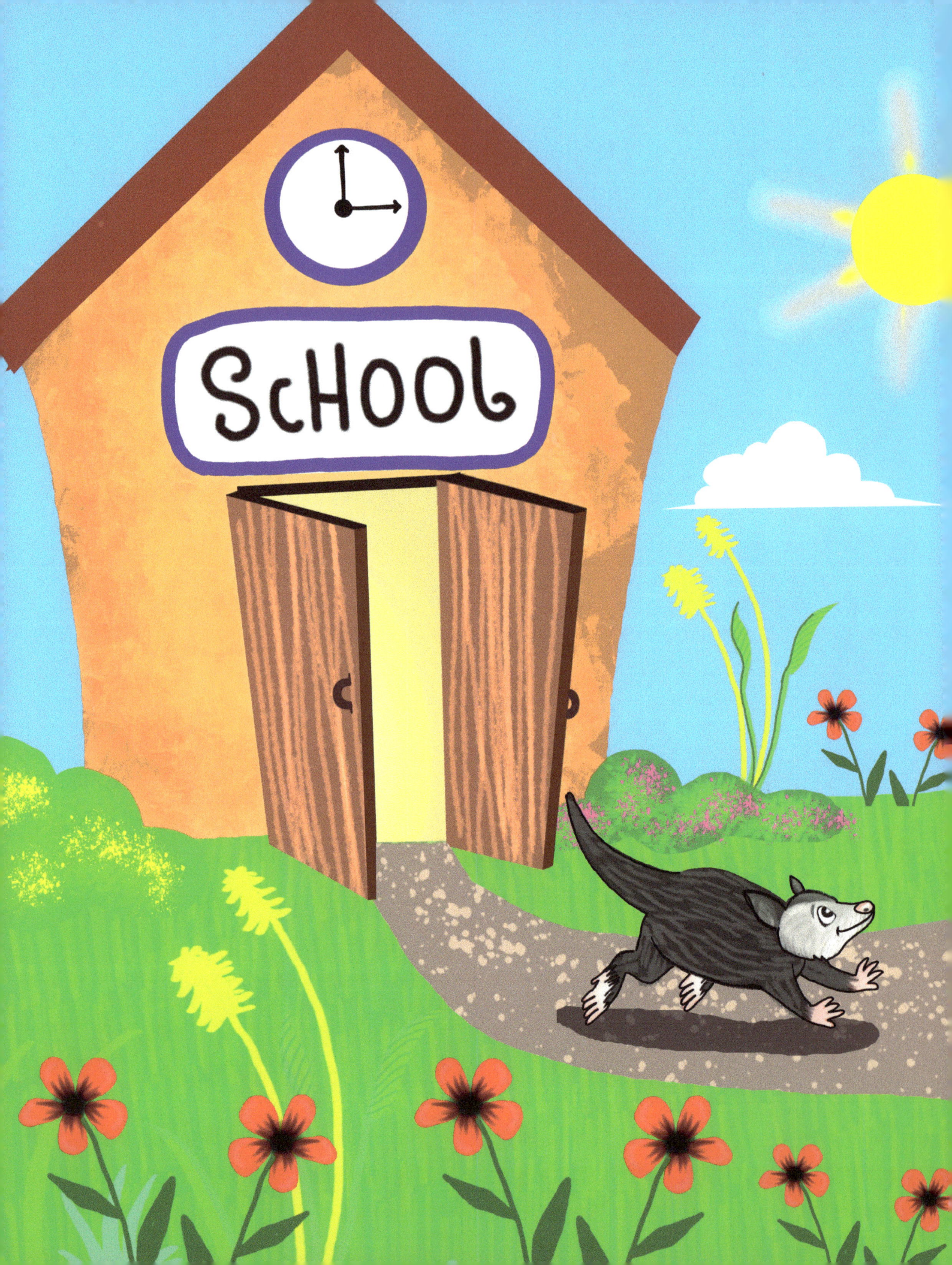

I take a deep breath
and stretch to the sky.
Moving my body helps
me to try.

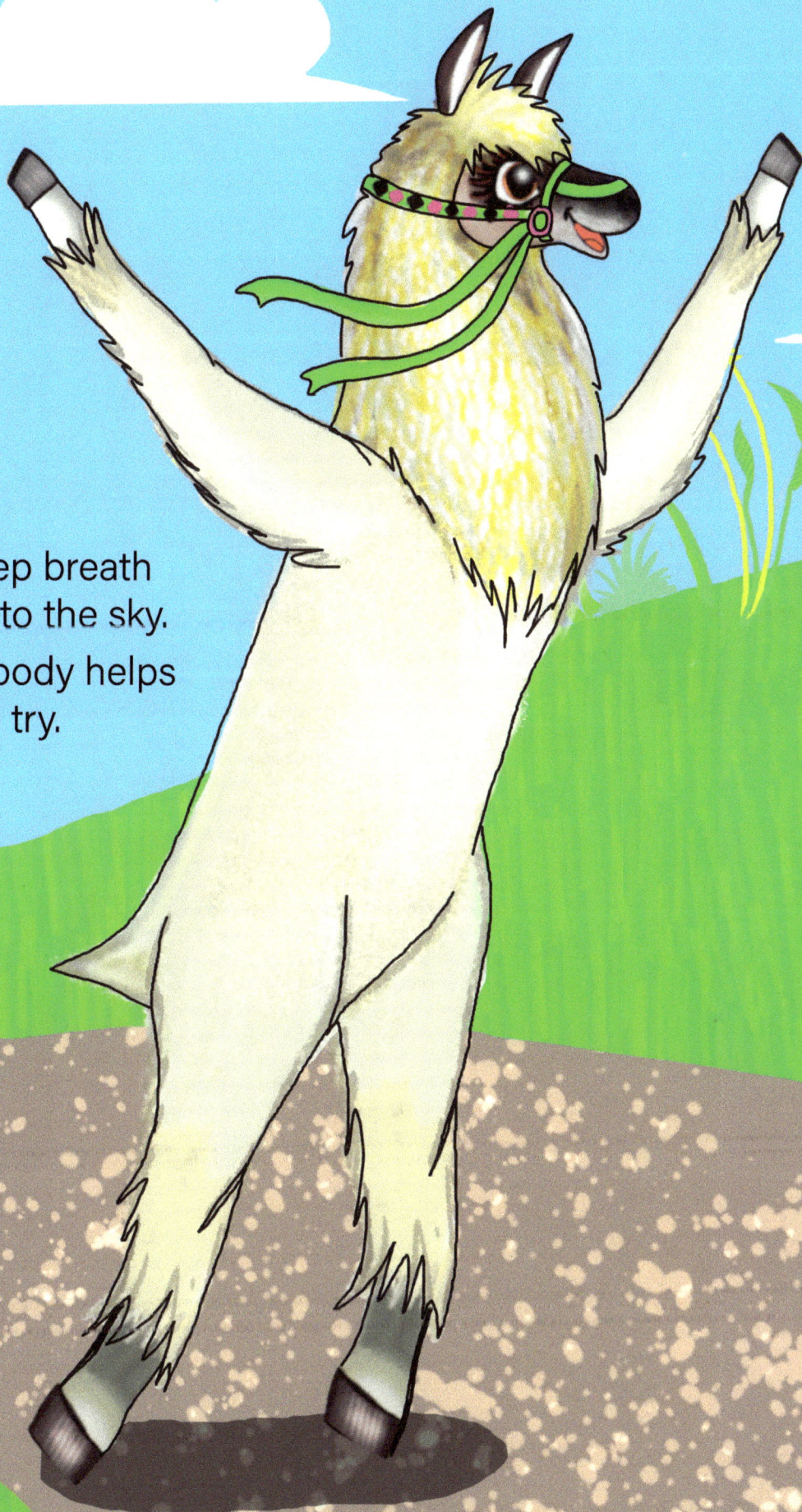

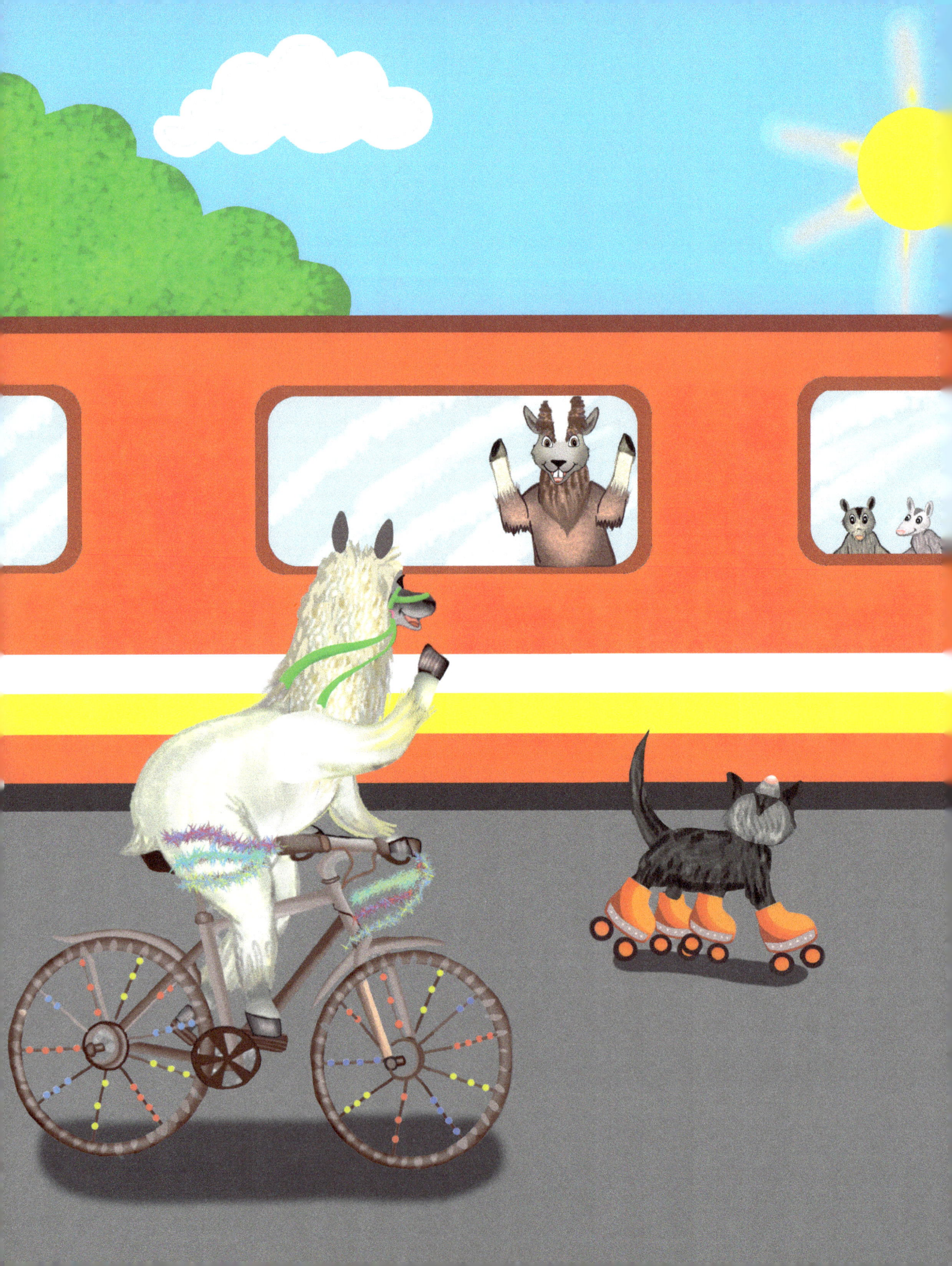

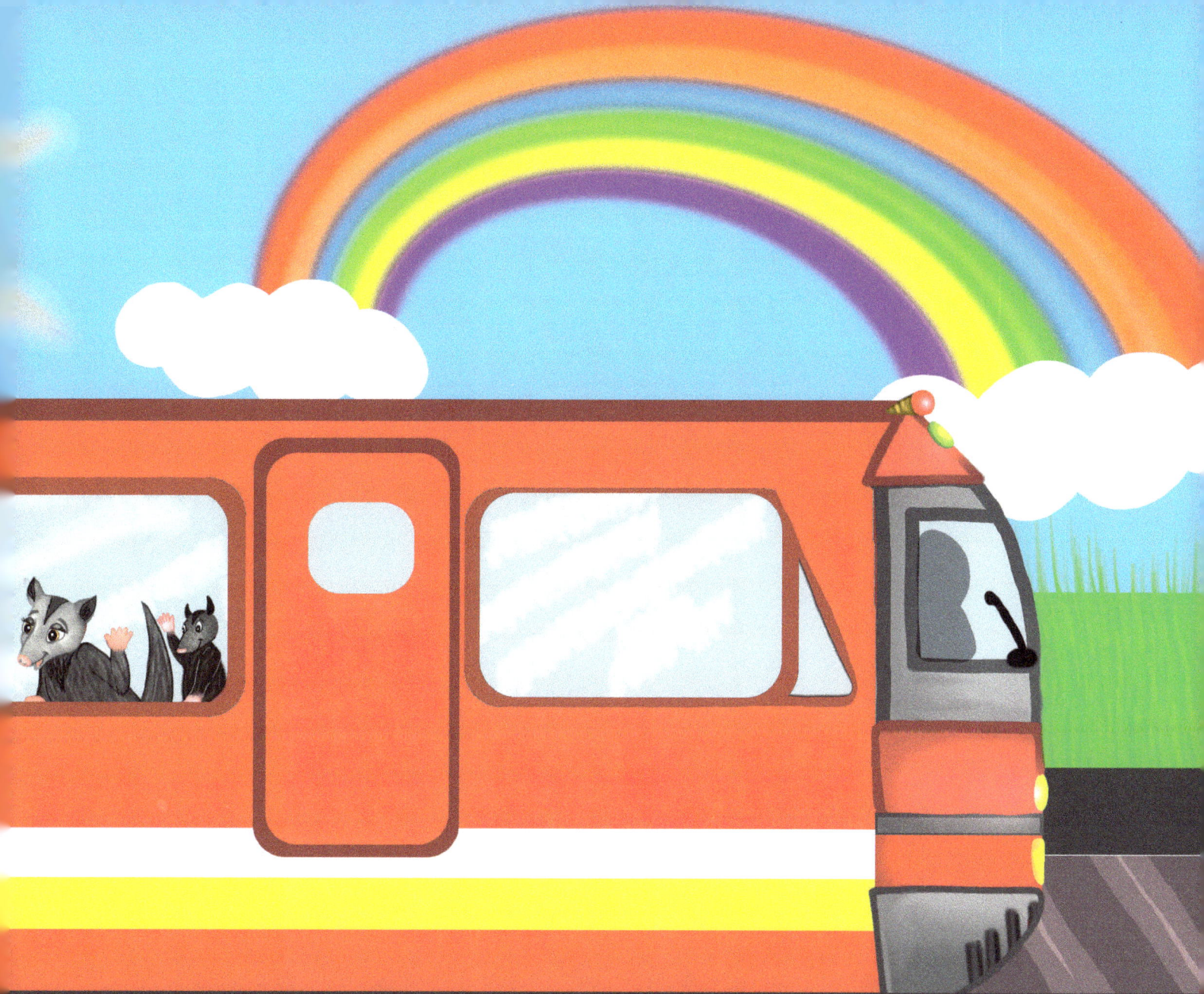

"Tell me, Llamas, how will you
move your body today?"

Author: Deborah Sharp Molchan, Ph.D.

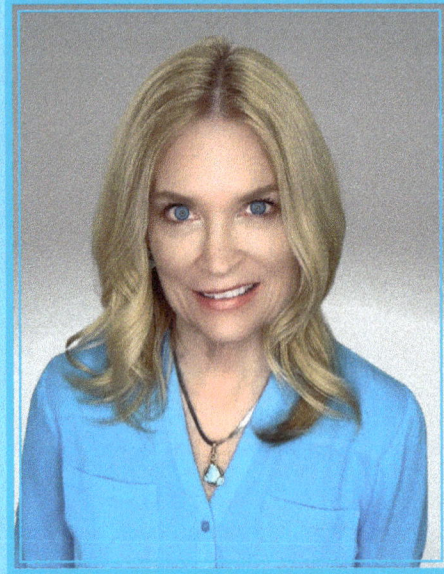

DR. MOLCHAN offers psychotherapy to clients in Uniontown and Pittsburgh, PA. Deborah is a Master's credentialed licensed psychologist. In 2013, Dr. Molchan completed her doctorate in psychology. As an adjunct professor, she taught graduate-level clinical psychology courses at Pennsylvania Western University and undergraduate psychology courses at Pennsylvania Western University and Pennsylvania State University. Deborah has presented to collegiate athletes at Westminster College, Moravian College, and local high school sports teams.

When Deborah is not working, she finds joy in various activities, including laughing with family and friends, skiing, golfing, sailing, running, and yoga. Her diverse interests, coupled with her years of clinical practice and research in psychology, fuel Dr. Molchan's creative process.

Illustrator: Emily Hercock

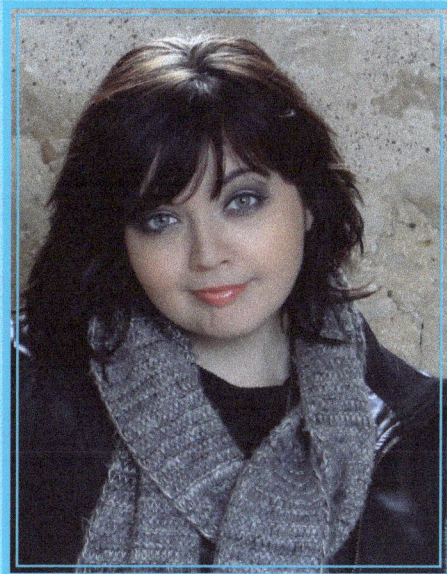

EMILY has worked as a freelance illustrator for nearly ten years, building her business from the ground up.

As a child, Emily could always be found with a pen and paper in her hand, drawing away at her latest artwork creation.

Emily never believed that she could make a career out of her hobby. But, with a lot of determination and hard work, she has been able to successfully turn her love of art into her own business.

Emily lives in the small, sleepy village of Watlington in the UK, where she resides with her husband, Michael, and thoroughly-mad cats, Rupert and Niko.

Author's Note to Parents, Caregivers, and Teachers

———◆———

Research confirms that physical activity helps children's brains focus and learn. The WHO (World Health Organization, 2022) recommends that children and adolescents exercise at a moderate to vigorous level for an average of 60 minutes daily and limit sedentary activities such as watching television and screen time. Parents, caregivers, and teachers can nurture children and adolescents to embrace exercise through example, setting appropriate limits on screen time, and shared family activities involving exercise, ideally in nature.

Teach children that a daily exercise habit prepares the mind for school work. Begin the day with habits of movement. Parents and caregivers may play movement games of skipping with children before leaving for school while singing, "Body motion is a great brain potion." Reminding children that vigorous physical activity prepares the brain for schoolwork is helpful.

Teachers are great at noticing when children's focus is waning. Frequently, a jumping jack break followed by slow breathing helps children regain focus. Fortunately, both adults and children benefit from a movement break.

Encourage children to run, jump, or skip before doing their homework. Body movement that increases our heart rate promotes the best conditions for attention, memory, and focus. Help your children set healthy limits with screen time and reinforce movement health by sharing observations such as, "You've been watching television for 20 minutes—time to move our bodies. Let's bike."

Be creative. On cold winter days, when an increased tendency to sit indoors may occur, take movement and exercise breaks after periods of sitting. Integrate exercise with sedentary activities like watching movies, taking breaks, pausing the show and marching in place, practicing yoga postures, or brisk walking or skipping around your house. Encourage children to take turns as Llama Locomotion Captains, leading the exercise breaks with their choice of movement practices.

When children make exercise a daily habit, they strengthen movement as a coping tool. And when parents, caregivers, and teachers embrace a playful attitude toward exercise, everyone benefits!

www.ingramcontent.com/pod-product-compliance
Lightning Source LLC
Chambersburg PA
CBHW041604260326
41914CB00011B/1379